# Coping with Schizophrenia

Professor Kevin Gournay CBE is a Registered Psychologist, Chartered Scientist and a Registered Nurse who is an Emeritus Professor at the Institute of Psychiatry, King's College London. He has many years of experience in contributing to the development of government policies in the UK and other countries, and in particular those that affect people with schizophrenia. He has also taught on this topic for health professionals in many countries across the world, and has worked for the World Health Organization. He has written numerous papers on the subject, including those based on his research. He continues his clinical work with people with schizophrenia and their families.

Dr Debbie Robson, RMN, BSc (Hons), MSc, PhD is a registered nurse who has a research, teaching and clinical role at the Institute of Psychiatry, King's College London and the South London and Maudsley NHS Foundation Trust. She has many years of experience in teaching professionals about the care and management of people with schizophrenia.

D0242599

# Overcoming Common Problems Series

*Selected titles*

A full list of titles is available from Sheldon Press,
36 Causton Street, London SW1P 4ST and on our website at
www.sheldonpress.co.uk

**Breast Cancer: Your treatment choices**
Dr Terry Priestman

**Cider Vinegar**
Margaret Hills

**Coeliac Disease: What you need to know**
Alex Gazzola

**Coping Successfully with Chronic Illness:
Your healing plan**
Neville Shone

**Coping Successfully with Shyness**
Margaret Oakes, Professor Robert Bor
and Dr Carina Eriksen

**Coping with Anaemia**
Dr Tom Smith

**Coping with Difficult Families**
Dr Jane McGregor and Tim McGregor

**Coping with Drug Problems in the Family**
Lucy Jolin

**Coping with Eating Disorders and Body Image**
Christine Craggs-Hinton

**Coping with Epilepsy**
Dr Pamela Crawford and Fiona Marshall

**Coping with Guilt**
Dr Windy Dryden

**Coping with Liver Disease**
Mark Greener

**Coping with Obsessive Compulsive Disorder**
Professor Kevin Gournay, Rachel Piper
and Professor Paul Rogers

**Coping with Schizophrenia**
Professor Kevin Gournay and Debbie Robson

**Depressive Illness – the Curse of the Strong**
Dr Tim Cantopher

**The Diabetes Healing Diet**
Mark Greener and Christine Craggs-Hinton

**Dying for a Drink**
Dr Tim Cantopher

**The Empathy Trap: Understanding Antisocial
Personalities**
Dr Jane McGregor and Tim McGregor

**Epilepsy: Complementary and alternative
treatments**
Dr Sallie Baxendale

**Fibromyalgia: Your Treatment Guide**
Christine Craggs-Hinton

**Hay Fever: How to beat it**
Dr Paul Carson

**The Heart Attack Survival Guide**
Mark Greener

**Helping Elderly Relatives**
Jill Eckersley

**The Holistic Health Handbook**
Mark Greener

**How to Come Out of Your Comfort Zone**
Dr Windy Dryden

**How to Eat Well When You Have Cancer**
Jane Freeman

**How to Stop Worrying**
Dr Frank Tallis

**The Irritable Bowel Diet Book**
Rosemary Nicol

**Living with Complicated Grief**
Professor Craig A. White

**Living with IBS**
Nuno Ferreira and David T. Gillanders

**Making Sense of Trauma: How to tell
your story**
Dr Nigel C. Hunt and Dr Sue McHale

**Overcoming Fear: With mindfulness**
Deborah Ward

**Overcoming Loneliness**
Alice Muir

**The Panic Workbook**
Dr Carina Eriksen, Professor Robert Bor
and Margaret Oakes

**Physical Intelligence: How to take charge
of your weight**
Dr Tom Smith

**The Self-Esteem Journal**
Alison Waines

**Transforming Eight Deadly Emotions
into Healthy Ones**
Dr Windy Dryden

**Treating Arthritis: The drug-free way**
Margaret Hills and Christine Horner

**Treating Arthritis: The supplements guide**
Julia Davies

**When Someone You Love Has Depression:
A handbook for family and friends**
Barbara Baker

Overcoming Common Problems

# Coping with Schizophrenia

PROFESSOR KEVIN GOURNAY
and
DR DEBBIE ROBSON

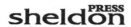

First published in Great Britain in 2014

Sheldon Press
36 Causton Street
London SW1P 4ST
www.sheldonpress.co.uk

Copyright © Professor Kevin Gournay and Dr Debbie Robson 2014

All rights reserved. No part of this book may be reproduced or
transmitted in any form or by any means, electronic or mechanical,
including photocopying, recording, or by any information storage and
retrieval system, without permission in writing from the publisher.

The authors and publisher have made every effort to ensure that the
external website and email addresses included in this book are correct and
up to date at the time of going to press. The authors and publisher are
not responsible for the content, quality or continuing accessibility of the
sites.

*British Library Cataloguing-in-Publication Data*
A catalogue record for this book is available from the British Library

ISBN 978–1–84709–264–9
eBook ISBN 978–1–84709–265–6

eBook by Fakenham Prepress Solutions, Fakenham, Norfolk NR21 8NN

Typeset by Fakenham Prepress Solutions, Fakenham, Norfolk NR21 8NN
First printed in Great Britain by Ashford Colour Press
Subsequently digitally reprinted in Great Britain

Produced on paper from sustainable forests

### From Kevin
*After the death of my father in 2010 I came to truly understand how families can provide more than any health professional in times of loss and hardship. Every living member of my father's family was present when we celebrated his life in a convivial occasion held at Charlton Athletic Football Club; I dedicate my part in this book to them.*

### From Debbie
*For Aimee and Scott, you make me proud and I never stop learning from you.*

### From Auz
*For my family who have always supported me. For my chosen sisters who help me feel like a better person. For my chosen brothers who accept me for who I am. And for my Constant Companion.*

### From Georgie
*For Christian, you are and always will be my hero.*

# Contents

# Foreword

There are many misunderstandings and myths concerning schizophrenia. It is frequently but incorrectly portrayed as a 'split' personality, and the person with the condition is seen as a Jekyll and Hyde character with the amoral wickedness of the latter. The label attracts a degree of fear and discrimination that is reflected in the isolation and exclusion of those with schizophrenia and their families, high rates of unemployment and suboptimal care and treatment of co-incidental physical ill health. The unpredictable and dangerous behaviour of a few has come to be the stigmata of all people with the condition, even though the reality is that they are far more likely to be the recipients of abuse and violence and of self-harm and suicide. Perhaps the worst myth of all is that it is impossible for the person affected to make any sensible decisions or to recover from the condition.

In *Coping with Schizophrenia*, Kevin Gournay and Debbie Robson provide much-needed information for those with schizophrenia and their families about the condition and the services and treatments that are available. At the heart of the book is a message of hope. Around half of those affected will experience a substantial recovery with still more achieving stability without further worsening. Furthermore, there is good evidence that treatment, particularly where given promptly early in the course of the disorder, reduces relapse and hospitalization. The use of medication is discussed in some detail, as befits the treatment that is still the most effective intervention for the symptoms of the condition, but it has to be taken over many months or even years after the acute episode has resolved. Although medication remains the mainstay of treatment, there has been a dramatic growth in the evidence for the benefit of talking treatments including cognitive behavioural therapy and family-focused interventions. These, particularly when offered alongside medication, dramatically reduce the frequency and severity of psychotic experiences and associated distress. Unfortunately, as the authors comment, these treatments are expensive, require skilled therapists and are less readily available than they should be, despite good evidence that they pay for themselves in terms of reduced relapse and reliance on expensive inpatient care.

While the overall message of the book is rightly optimistic, a great deal of attention is directed at the shocking physical health outcomes of people who suffer from psychotic disorders. Those with a diagnosis of schizophrenia are at increased risk of physical ill health, including heart and respiratory diseases, diabetes and some cancers, dying some 20 years earlier than their contemporaries in the general population. Much of this risk is preventable as it is linked to behaviours that can be changed, as for example a fatty diet, tobacco smoking, excessive alcohol and inadequate exercise, all of which are more often found among people suffering from schizophrenia. For example, it has been estimated that 60 per cent of sufferers smoke tobacco, compared with 20 per cent of the general population, and that nearly half of all the tobacco consumed in England is by people with mental health problems. A similar story can be recounted for poor diet, low exercise and obesity. But in addition to this, the risk behaviours and associated poor health are likely to be overlooked by the health service. Psychiatrists and psychiatric nurses tend to regard physical health monitoring and treatment as the business of the patient's General Practitioner, while GPs and other non-psychiatric professionals either do not see the patients or if they do, tend to focus on the mental health problem and miss the physical complaint or assume that the patient would be incapable of understanding or following the health advice they would ordinarily give to a non-mentally ill patient. Of course, most good GPs would be horrified to think they could be capable of such obvious neglect, and there are efforts to tackle the shortcomings of the existing divisions between mental and physical health care. But this can only go so far. Ultimately, as in medicine generally, a good part of the success of preventive interventions relies on the individual's awareness of the risk and his or her belief that something can be done about the risk. The strength of this book is that it provides people with schizophrenia and their families with the information they need, enabling better self-care and empowering help and advice seeking.

Professor Tom K. J. Craig
Institute of Psychiatry
Kings College London

# Acknowledgements

We would like to thank Auz Thompson and Georgie Wakefield for so generously sharing their experiences of schizophrenia in this book.

This book would not have been written, but for the experiences of Debbie and Kevin in their years of working with people with schizophrenia, their families and carers. While our experience has in many ways been positive, because of the numerous individuals who have either recovered or achieved great relief from distress and suffering, we have also been struck by the way, for others, professional care and treatment has either not been provided or provided at suboptimal levels. These collective experiences have led to this book and we must therefore acknowledge countless people with schizophrenia who have provided our motivation.

We also wish to thank those professional colleagues, too numerous to mention, who have provided us with education, training, clinical supervision, mentorship and support. We must also mention many others, in the voluntary sector, journalism and in areas far removed from mental health care, who have also been sources of inspiration.

# Note to the reader

This is not a medical book and is not intended to replace advice from your doctor. Consult your pharmacist or doctor if you believe you have any of the symptoms described, and if you think you might need medical help.

# Introduction

When our publisher asked us to write this book, we were very pleased to provide something that might be of potential benefit to the, literally, hundreds of thousands of people in the UK with schizophrenia, their families and their carers. Like ourselves, our publisher was aware that, compared with the vast amount of scientific literature on the topic, there was very little in the way of self-help material for those affected by this illness. We were also aware that a book such as this might contribute to the public understanding of schizophrenia and, in turn, serve to reduce the tremendous stigma associated with this and other mental health problems.

At the time of completing this book (at the end of 2012 and the beginning of 2013) a report by the Schizophrenia Commission, chaired by Professor Sir Robin Murray, FRS, was published and aptly titled *The Abandoned Illness*. The commission was set up by the national charity Rethink Mental Illness because of the disquiet among people with schizophrenia and others affected by the condition. Later in the book we will provide more information about the findings of the commission, published in a report in 2012, which we commend and suggest you read in its entirety. Also of note in 2012, the Royal College of Psychiatrists conducted an audit of services and published its findings later in the year in the form of a report.

Before we began writing, we decided that we had three overall aims. First, we wished to provide as much information as possible about schizophrenia, believing that all too often, information about mental health problems is deemed as the property of health professionals and can only be shared very selectively with those without the necessary professional background and training. On the contrary, our belief is that information truly is power, and that people with schizophrenia and all those interested should be provided with as much information as possible about the illness, because an understanding of a condition is the first step in self-help.

Having set the scene, our second aim was to provide information about the services that are available and to provide a realistic picture of all treatment and care options. In considering this, we were confronted with the far from ideal situation that exists in the UK today. On the one hand, we know that there is much that can be done by way of treatment and care to reduce the distress and suffering caused by schizophrenia. On the other hand, we also know that the reality is that, for a variety of reasons, many people are not offered the best available care and treatment options.

Our third aim was to provide advice about self-help to those with schizophrenia, their families, carers and friends. We thought long and hard about the range of potential self-help topics, and considered what advice other self-help books have previously offered. We therefore wrote a long list of topics: everything from how to access legal advice to how to cope with voices (auditory hallucinations). One topic stood out as being of vital importance – how to maintain the best possible physical health.

Why did we arrive at that decision? The answer is simple – on average, people with schizophrenia live about 15 years less than the general population but, more positively, we know that this need not be the case as there is a great deal that can be done to prevent the illnesses that are common among people with schizophrenia. We have given detailed advice on a range of health topics and also cover practical matters, such as how to deal with obstacles that may prevent reasonable access to the interventions needed. We have devoted a very large section of this book to self-help information. For this we offer no apology. We say, look at the facts – people with schizophrenia, on average, unnecessarily lose many years of life.

A final thought regarding our third aim of providing appropriate self-help advice is the question of how we could most effectively convey this information. The answer was obvious – ask those who know best. We have therefore enlisted the expert advice and co-authorship of two people: one who has schizophrenia and one carer. They will tell their stories and say what has worked for them.

## What's in a name?

We have thought long and hard about the most acceptable term to use with regard to people with schizophrenia who receive services. Throughout this book we will generally use the term 'people with schizophrenia'. However, there are occasions when there is a need to use a word or a term in relation to treatments and care processes.

Currently, some mental health services use the term 'patient' to describe such an individual. Some organizations devoted to giving a voice to people who use services prefer the word 'survivor'. Psychotherapists and psychologists often (but not always) prefer the word 'client' and, of course, many use the word 'patient'.

In keeping with our philosophy of basing this book on evidence, we decided that we should look to studies conducted by a range of people with interest in the topic. Unsurprisingly in our view, we found that if you ask people with schizophrenia and their carers their preferred form of address, there is a wide range of responses. Overall, however, it appears that 'patient' is the preferred term, particularly when used within the context of people receiving care from mental health professionals, including social workers and occupational therapists, who (with other groups of people) prefer 'client'.

We have therefore decided to use 'patient' throughout the book, when appropriate. With regard to our personal preference, although we understand that 'patient' may be used in a way that indicates an unfair balance of power between the professional and the individual, for a registered health professional the word implies a considerable emphasis on a duty of care and also indicates the importance of working within a moral and ethical framework of the highest standard. Finally, schizophrenia is undoubtedly an illness, like cancer, high blood pressure or diabetes. People with these physical illnesses are called, and call themselves, patients. Therefore, patient it is!

With apologies to those who prefer another form of address, a last word. In our opinion, what is important in a book such as this is conveying as much information as possible to patients and families and carers; we truly believe that information is power.

# Part 1
# SIGNS, SYMPTOMS AND DIAGNOSIS

# 1

# What is schizophrenia?

## History

The word schizophrenia was first used by the psychiatrist Eugen Bleuler just over one hundred years ago. The word, literally translated from the Greek, means 'splitting of the mind', hence the incorrect belief among many that people with schizophrenia have a 'split personality'. This was not Bleuler's intent and, even then, he realized that schizophrenia was a highly complex condition involving personality, thinking, memory and perception.

Before that, others realized that schizophrenia was different from dementia, intellectual disabilities and the common mental health problems such as depression and anxiety, and that it appears in many shapes and forms. Over the years there have been various attempts to classify schizophrenia. The current classifications can be found in the American Psychiatric Association's *Diagnostic and Statistical Manual of Mental Disorders*, 5th edition (DSM-5) and the World Health Organization's *International Classification of Diseases*, revision 10 (ICD-10). The classifications used now are still controversial and international experts disagree with one another. However, what seems to be clear is that schizophrenia is probably best thought of as an 'umbrella' term to describe a number of conditions that may manifest themselves in quite different ways and require differing approaches to treatment and care.

## Signs, symptoms and diagnosis

Over the years there have been a number of controversies about diagnosis. Thirty years ago, many psychiatrists disagreed about whether a particular individual had schizophrenia. It was also true to say that the diagnosis was often made after the individual had spent many years in contact with mental health professionals without their problems being recognized. Although the situation is now far from perfect, mental health professionals across the world are now in much greater agreement about what constitutes a schizophrenic illness. Of considerable importance, many countries now have programmes dedicated to improving diagnosis, so that treatments may begin earlier in the disease. There is certainly accumulating evidence that early intervention is beneficial for long-term outcomes.

Schizophrenia presents in various forms or subtypes, and even within the subtypes there is considerable variation between individuals. Broadly speaking, one of the most accepted ways of looking at signs and symptoms is to divide and classify them as positive, negative and cognitive. When professionals talk about 'positive' symptoms they do not mean symptoms that are helpful or provide a benefit, they are referring to psychological experiences that are added to or exaggerated in someone's personality. 'Negative' refers to symptoms that are deficits or reductions of normal emotional responses. 'Cognitive' refers to how we think and process information. Examples of some of the symptoms of schizophrenia and how they are classified are given in Table 1.

It is worth noting that people with schizophrenia commonly have other mental health problems. It is important that these are identified and appropriately treated; it is sadly all too common to

**Table 1 Symptoms of schizophrenia**

| Type of symptom | Symptom |
|---|---|
| Positive | Delusions |
| | Hallucinations |
| | Behavioural changes |
| Negative | Apathy |
| | Blunting of emotions |
| | Incongruity of emotions/responses |
| | Reduction in speech |
| | Social withdrawal |
| | Reduction in social performance |
| Cognitive | Problems with working memory |
| | Poor executive functioning |
| | Inability to sustain attention |

see with people with schizophrenia experiencing various anxieties, fears and phobias that are not being addressed by mental health professionals (see 'Other mental health problems' in this chapter).

## Positive symptoms

### Delusions

There are a number of definitions of a delusion. Indeed, if one looks at the books written about schizophrenia, some authors have written literally thousands of words in their attempt to tell us what delusions are. One definition that we prefer is simple: a false belief that is impervious to reason or logic and has no evidence to support it. However, the issue of context needs to be taken into account when applying this definition. One obvious example is that of spiritual and religious beliefs. Many religious beliefs appear to have little or no hard evidence to support them and are regarded as a matter of faith. It would therefore be ridiculous to regard all people of faith as delusional. Likewise, there are certain beliefs held within certain cultures that appear to others not within that culture to be irrational and illogical and also without any evidence base. What might therefore distinguish a delusion from a religious or cultural belief? This perhaps might best be explained by an example:

> Peter is a 24-year-old man who grew up in a village in Somerset. He attended the local Church of England service every Sunday morning with his family and went to a church school. Throughout his childhood and adolescence Peter took part in a number of Christian activities and was always proud to say that he was a committed Christian. At 18 years of age he left home to go to university, where he studied physics and obtained a good degree. While at university he joined the Society of Christian Students, where he often discussed how he approached what appeared to be an incompatibility between hard science and faith. Indeed, Peter left university saying that the more he learned about the universe, the stronger his faith had actually become.
>
> Shortly after leaving university, Peter encountered a number of significant life stresses, including the sudden death of his mother. He gradually became more withdrawn and depressed, and although he continued to work he did little else – even neglecting to attend his usual Sunday service. After a while Peter told his father that the reason for his withdrawal was his belief that there were people watching him and that he would need to wait until they told him what to do with his life. It also seemed clear that Peter believed that those watching

him had told him that if he continued to go to church 'something bad' would happen to his father and the rest of his family. Peter eventually went to an accident and emergency department in a state of panic because he felt that 'these people' were pursuing him. The hospital represented a place of safety. He was referred to the duty mental health nurse, who spoke to Peter for about an hour and a half. She found that Peter's beliefs about 'these people' were completely fixed and despite reassurance that he would be safe he continued to feel under very serious threat.

Following a short admission to hospital and treatment with medication and cognitive behavioural therapy (see Chapter 8) Peter eventually made a good recovery from his illness, which was diagnosed as schizophrenia. Several months later, when he had returned to normal function and resumed going to church and, indeed, was making plans to get married to his long-term girlfriend, he told his community psychiatric nurse that he remembered how he was at the height of his illness and how everything had seemed like a bad dream. He was also able to say that he was, at the time, completely convinced that others were in some way controlling him and that nothing that anyone could have said or done would have convinced him otherwise. He said that obtaining insight into his illness and understanding that his convictions were part of that illness took him several months. These beliefs, which he now recognized as delusions, did not simply go away. They very slowly diminished in strength and intensity until they were no longer present.

## Hallucinations

Hallucinations are best defined as sensory experiences for which there is no external stimulus. All five senses – taste, sight, touch, smell and hearing – can be affected. It is worth emphasizing that hallucinations are not necessarily a sign of mental illness and there is a wide variety of research that shows that hallucinations occur in many people who are in good mental health. Indeed, we have all probably experienced hallucinations – just before sleep or on waking up (hypnagogic or hypnopompic hallucinations, respectively). They may also occur under extremes of stress and tiredness.

The most common form of hallucination in schizophrenia is hearing voices. These sometimes take the form of a commentary on what the person is doing or what is happening around them and at other times may come in the form of commands.

Sometimes the voices are pleasant in tone or content but they can be critical, and very distressing as a result. Many people with schizophrenia realize that the voices are not real but are part of their illness, while others perceive them to be real and if they are particularly critical, serve to compound the person's distress. It is therefore very important that the professionals or family members around a person with schizophrenia take the time and trouble to understand the nature and content of the voices. As we will see later, an understanding of the voices is the first step in developing a coping strategy.

### Thoughts and thinking problems

One feature of some but not all cases of schizophrenia is thought disorders and problems of thinking. All of us have problems with thinking, every day of our lives. Just recall those occasions when your mind 'goes blank' or where you lose your concentration – or simply when your mind suddenly jumps from one topic to another. Some people experience more of these problems than others. However, for most of us these problems of thoughts and thinking do not interfere with our everyday lives and pose no real problems in our interaction with others. In schizophrenia, problems of thinking may be very prominent and cause great disruption of all aspects of life.

The main problem for the affected person sometimes concerns attention and concentration. These problems are often connected with the great distraction caused by hallucinations, or by the pre-occupation with a delusional idea. People with schizophrenia can experience thought blocking, where a train of thinking suddenly stops. The individual may then pause and continue with a train of thought on a completely different subject. American psychiatrist Dr Nancy Andreasen has catalogued some of the thought problems encountered in schizophrenia:

*Derailment*  Wandering off of the point during the free flow of conversation.

*Tangentiality*  Answering questions that are off the point.

*Incoherence*  Breakdown of the relationships of words within a sentence so that the sentence no longer makes sense.

*Loss of goal*  Failure to reach a conclusion or achieve a point.

Dr Andreasen also describes unusual uses of language – for example, people with schizophrenia often invent new words (neologisms) to describe a particular, novel experience.

## Changes in behaviour

Delusions and hallucinations may lead to behavioural changes. However, behaviour such as agitation and overactivity may occur without any apparent connection to delusions or hallucinations. The overactivity seen in some types of schizophrenia can lead to exhaustion, weight loss and sometimes serious physical illness.

Among the other behavioural changes seen in schizophrenia are increases in fluid drinking and food intake. Although these may be connected with the side effects of medication (some medications cause an increase in appetite) they should be investigated by the patient's GP.

## Negative symptoms

### Apathy

One of the changes that family members often observe in the early stages of the illness is a change in interest and enthusiasm for pastimes and hobbies that have previously given great enjoyment. The person will often describe 'losing interest'.

### Blunting of emotions

Some people with schizophrenia experience 'blunting' of emotions and lack of emotional response to events that would normally make the person sad, happy or excited.

### Incongruity of emotions

This describes the way in which some people with schizophrenia react inappropriately in their mood and reactions to external events. For example, on hearing news of a family member who has died or suffered serious illness, a person with schizophrenia may react by laughing or giggling. Likewise, quite ordinary interactions may lead to outbursts of anger or irritability.

### Reduction in speech

This may be an early sign of the illness but is common at any stage. It is sometimes difficult to keep a conversation going because the person shows what is often described as 'impoverished' speech or verbal responses.

### Social withdrawal

People with schizophrenia will often withdraw from interactions with other people and can often become extremely reclusive. Even if they find themselves in social situations they will withdraw and be uncommunicative.

### Reduction in social performance

An early sign of schizophrenia may be a change in social performance. Thus, a person who has previously performed well socially begins to show poor social skills. This may be demonstrated in problems at work or with peers in social groups at college or university.

## Cognitive symptoms

In addition to the impact positive symptoms and thought disorder have on concentration and thinking, further cognitive impairments often interfere with a person's ability to lead a productive and independent life. These symptoms are usually present before the onset of the illness and before a person receives treatment.

### Problems with working memory

The ability to use information immediately after reading or hearing something, and making decisions based on that information, is often impaired in people with schizophrenia.

### Poor executive functioning

Executive functions include the capacity to formulate goals, to plan, organize and carry out a particular behaviour fully and effectively, and to monitor and self-correct behaviour. Doing simple tasks such as shopping for groceries or following a recipe can often be difficult. Being able to make choices when more than one option is presented can also present difficulty. Because poor executive functioning may lead to difficulties in censoring thoughts and behaviour, the person may talk out loud inappropriately in social situations.

### Problems with maintaining attention

People with schizophrenia may be easily distracted and find it difficult to begin and remain focused on any task or even a thought. Watching a TV programme all the way through or reading a book from beginning to end may take a huge amount of effort.

### Other mental health problems

Up to one-quarter of people with schizophrenia also have depression, and many others experience anxiety, phobias and obsessions. These problems are also extremely common in the general population and there is no reason why people with schizophrenia should be less affected. As we have already noted, mental health professionals can pay insufficient attention to other mental health problems in people with schizophrenia, which is particularly sad, as we know that when these problems are appropriately targeted with psychological therapies considerable benefits may be obtained.

## Persistent and recurrent schizophrenia

At the most severe end of the spectrum are people who continue to have symptoms of schizophrenia and experience intermittent worsening, regardless of the treatment that they receive. This group of people has often been treated with a wide range of medications, with little effect. There is now evidence that the addition of a psychological treatment such as cognitive behavioural therapy (CBT) leads to a great improvement in function. A study by van der Gaag and colleagues in the Netherlands showed that people who received CBT experienced twice as many days of normal social functioning than those who received treatment as usual (van der Gaag *et al.* 2011).

# 2

# Causes of schizophrenia

What then causes schizophrenia? The simple answer – probably a combination of factors. While schizophrenia is a disease of the brain, we also know that our genetic makeup is central to whether or not we will develop the disease. The environment also plays a part. This chapter reviews the evidence.

## Genetics

Although there has been a vast amount of research into the condition, and our understanding of the brain has improved dramatically with the advent of new technologies, there is still much we do not know regarding the causes of schizophrenia. Although it has been clear for many years that most forms of schizophrenia may have a genetic basis, the more we learn about genes the more we find that there is no single genetic explanation. You can therefore discard the thought that a gene of schizophrenia is about to be discovered.

We have known for many years that having a first-degree relative with schizophrenia increases the risk of developing the condition. A number of studies of identical twins have shown that, even when separated at birth and brought up in different environments, the likelihood of both twins having schizophrenia is substantial. A couple of decades ago, when new technologies allowed us to research the human genome, some scientists thought that the discovery of the 'schizophrenia gene' was just around the corner. However, although we have discovered that there are many genes involved in the causation of the condition, there are still a number of unknowns. For example, there is no explanation for why one person with the genes known to be associated with the condition manifests a range of signs and symptoms, while another person with the same genes appears to have no mental health problems. Even more intriguing, the genes associated with schizophrenia in one generation may be passed to someone in the next generation who shows signs and symptoms of another illness, such as bipolar disorder (previously known as manic depression).

## Stress vulnerability

Some 35 years ago, a psychologist and a psychiatrist (Professor Bonnie Spring and Profession Joseph Zubin) from the USA put forward a theory that has now become very influential in the way that we see schizophrenia and other psychotic illnesses. Essentially, the model proposes that some people are genetically vulnerable to developing schizophrenic-type illnesses and that these illnesses may be triggered by stress. The commonly cited stresses include developmental factors, including traumatic childhood events, social deprivation (particularly in early adult life) and, later on, physical stresses placed on the body such as substance abuse and, possibly, nutritional factors.

Once the illness has been triggered, the model also proposes that if current rather than past stress factors can be identified – such as poor social support, isolation, relationship problems and so on – it may be possible to influence the course of the illness by reducing these stresses. One important feature of the model is that the individual may be able to take an active role in reducing their vulnerability to stress and thereby reduce the severity of their illness. People who make a reasonable recovery from an episode of illness may then be able to recognize how to reduce stress in the future and thus prevent relapse.

## Drugs and alcohol

The past two decades have seen a massive increase in the use of illicit drugs in society. For example, cocaine, which at one time was the drug of choice for only the rich, has now become available at prices much lower than a few drinks in a pub. The use of other street drugs, such as heroin, has also increased; it is now being used by hundreds of thousands of people in the UK. There are various estimates for the use of ecstasy; many say that half a million ecstasy tablets are consumed every week in the UK. Add this to the array of 'legal highs' and a range of other 'uppers' and 'downers'. Illicit drug use in this country is a complex and all-consuming phenomenon.

In addition to street drugs there is also a steady supply, from the Internet, of prescription drugs known to be addictive – for example, the benzodiazepines, including diazepam (Valium) and lorazepam (Ativan). All of these drugs have important implications for people with schizophrenia. However, the drug linked most often with schizophrenia is cannabis and particularly the stronger varieties known as 'skunk'.

## What is important about the use of street/non-prescribed drugs?

First, it seems clear that stimulant drugs such as cocaine and amphetamines ('speed') can cause anyone to develop symptoms characteristic of schizophrenia, including feelings of persecution, high levels of excitement, outbursts of aggression and so on. In people with schizophrenia, taking these drugs is likely to greatly increase their level of illness and add to the symptoms they already have. It also seems clear that many illicit drugs (but particularly skunk) can cause some individuals to develop schizophrenia when, had they not taken the drug, they would have remained well. It is thought that there is a proportion of the population vulnerable to the development of schizophrenia following drug-taking. In all probability, this is owing to a genetic predisposition.

The combination of drug-taking and mental illness is now deemed one of the largest single problems confronting mental health professionals, and the terms 'dual diagnosis' and 'co-morbidity' have been used to describe those with a combination of drug problems and schizophrenia.

Alcohol is also a potential problem, and its prolonged use may of course lead to feelings of paranoia and other symptoms. Indeed, it is common to find that people who use illicit drugs also consume large quantities of alcohol. The results of surveys conducted in the UK and other countries in the Western world show that the dual-diagnosis population tends to consume not one but several drugs. Thus there are individuals who use cannabis on a daily basis and occasionally cocaine, heroin or other street drugs, and also consume alcohol.

The picture becomes even more complicated when taking into account the possibility that some individuals take drugs to alleviate the symptoms of mental illness. For example, cannabis is commonly used to decrease feelings of anxiety, and many people with schizophrenia say that the side effects of medications used to treat their schizophrenia cause them such distress that they use street drugs to combat them.

Overall, what we have is a very complicated picture of the way in which illicit drugs, alcohol and schizophrenia interact. The message seems clear: people with schizophrenia should avoid taking any drugs not prescribed for them and should, ideally, abstain from alcohol. That said, this recommendation appears to be unrealistic in many cases. For example, someone with schizophrenia who is at university may find it very difficult to avoid the offer of a 'joint'. Likewise, someone living in a culture where cannabis use is not only widespread but generally endorsed by that culture as positive will also find it difficult to resist.

Young people (the group most vulnerable to schizophrenia) are living in a world where cheap alcohol and street drugs are available in a steady 24-hour supply. While mental health professionals do what they can to deal with the problems of dual diagnosis or co-morbidity, the solution to the problem probably lies in the hands of society rather than mental health services.

## Childhood adversity

Childhood adversity and trauma have long been associated with an increased risk of developing psychosis (the positive symptoms of schizophrenia). By adversity and trauma we mean abuse, be it sexual, physical or emotional. It also refers to other serious life events such as parental separation and loss, as well as neglect, bullying and victimization. Professor Richard Bentall and colleagues from Liverpool University, in collaboration with researchers at Maastricht University in the Netherlands, have recently reviewed the findings of studies relating to this subject conducted over a 30-year period (Varase *et al.* 2012). They found that children who had experienced any type of trauma before the age of 16 were approximately three times more likely to become psychotic compared with children who had not experienced such adversity. Unsurprisingly, those who were severely traumatized as children were at greater risk of developing psychosis later in life.

## The role of dopamine

Genetic and environmental factors such as stress, drugs, alcohol or childhood adversity may influence the amount of the neurotransmitter dopamine in the brain, one of the chemicals involved in the passage of information between different nerve cells (neurones). Too much dopamine in a particular part of the brain is thought to be related to the positive symptoms of schizophrenia, whereas too little dopamine in another part is thought to be related to the negative symptoms.

Several other neurotransmitters are thought to be involved in the development and maintenance of symptoms, and the excess of dopamine may itself be a reaction to an as yet unknown cause. Our brain releases dopamine if something exciting happens to us, but it also releases it when something stressful or unexpected happens and also when we anticipate something. Dopamine is thus involved in the normal process of assigning meaning and importance to events. It teaches the brain to carry on being interested in something.

Exactly how an increased amount of dopamine accounts for delusional and hallucinatory experiences is still not entirely clear, despite the fact that scientists have been studying the role of dopamine and psychosis for over 50 years. The best understanding we have of this comes from the work of Professor Shitij Kapur at the Institute of Psychiatry, Kings College London, who has developed an interesting working model that brings together what we know about what is going on in the brains of people with schizophrenia, how they make sense of their world and how antipsychotic medication can influence the experience of symptoms (Kapur 2003).

There is wide-ranging evidence that people with untreated schizophrenia have an excess of dopamine in their brain – their brain is releasing too much of it. This changes the way dopamine works, so that things that happen in everyday life that should be of no significance become highly important. People who are psychotic have a tendency to see meaning and significance in external events and pay attention to internal thoughts and bodily sensations that tend to go unnoticed by people who do not have the condition. When people recount their initial experiences of the onset of the illness, and when they are in a state of relapse, they often talk of having a heightened awareness of all their senses – sounds, colours, smells, touch and taste are more acute. The world around them seems to be changing in some way and they may start to become fascinated by things that are trivial to others. For example, in Chapter 11, Georgie tells the story of her youngest son Christian, who developed schizophrenia at the age of 16. During the very early stages of his illness he became fascinated by the patterns on his clothes, believing that this fascination somehow affected his concentration at work. He eventually threw away all his patterned clothes.

Staying with Professor Kapur's framework, it is suggested that antipsychotic medications reduce the amount of dopamine in the brain, thereby reducing the importance and significance of the meanings people attach to external and internal experiences. A positive outcome of this new framework is that we are moving away from the either/or approach to drug and psychological treatments and seeing the importance of combining both approaches.

# 3

# Impact and outcome
# of schizophrenia

## How common is schizophrenia?

There are now literally dozens of studies from across the world that
have examined the prevalence and incidence of schizophrenia.
Prevalence is the total number of cases of a disease in a given population at a specific time, whereas incidence is, strictly speaking,
defined as the number of new cases of a specific disease occurring
during a certain period. Usually, incidence figures refer to lifetime.
Prevalence rates are therefore lower than incidence rates.

An interesting finding from these studies is that there has been
disagreement on diagnosis between even the most distinguished
experts and, importantly for people with schizophrenia and their
families, all the studies have shown that the diagnosis of schizophrenia is often much delayed. This leads to lost opportunities with
respect to providing effective treatment.

There is general agreement that schizophrenia affects about 7 in
1000 of the adult population at any one time. The World Health
Organization (WHO) states that schizophrenia affects 25 million
people worldwide. It also says that more than 50 per cent of persons
with schizophrenia are not receiving appropriate care and 90 per
cent of people with untreated schizophrenia are to be found in
developing countries.

Although schizophrenia can develop at any age, most cases begin
before the age of 25. However, the type and form of schizophrenic
illness varies with age of onset. Men tend to develop schizophrenia
slightly earlier than women.

## Physical problems

All the studies of schizophrenia conducted in large populations
demonstrate that people with schizophrenia are at much greater risk

of other health problems, notably cardiovascular and respiratory problems. Also, people with schizophrenia (possibly because of the nature of their illness) are more likely to acquire communicable diseases such as human immunodeficiency virus (HIV), hepatitis C and tuberculosis. People with schizophrenia have a much higher rate of diabetes and this seems to be caused by a combination of medication effects and unknown physical factors. The increased risk of diabetes was well established before the introduction of antipsychotic drugs, and researchers continue to investigate this association. See Chapter 13 for more about schizophrenia and health.

## Suicide

We thought long and hard about the inclusion of this subject in a book aimed at people with schizophrenia and their families. One of our principal aims is to inspire hope for all those affected by this condition and although we concluded that we could not totally avoid the topic of suicide we did not wish to add to the distress of some readers. Nevertheless, the subject of suicide is important because, in our opinion, although people with schizophrenia have a much greater risk of suicide than the general population, and suicide is a very common cause of death in people with schizophrenia, we also believe that effective treatment and care will greatly reduce this ultimate tragedy.

It is important to note that studies have recently shown that the greatest suicide risk occurs in the first 7 days after discharge from inpatient care and this is therefore the time when mental health professionals – and indeed families – need to be vigilant for signs of distress, despair or hopelessness. A feeling of hopelessness is a very important indicator of suicide and any complaints of hopelessness should be taken very seriously by anyone coming into contact with a person with schizophrenia.

# Outcomes

## Can you recover?

A number of studies from various countries have followed people with schizophrenia for many years following their diagnosis – several for more than 20 years, including two studies in the USA and one study in Switzerland that followed up people for more than 30 years.

These studies have shown that although a significant minority go on to suffer schizophrenia in a severe and chronic form, more positively, up to one-quarter of cases demonstrate complete recovery. Also, nearly half of those followed up had either completely recovered or only exhibited mild problems that did not interfere with community living. Even in the group who continued to have symptoms, up to 75 per cent were deemed to be stable after they had been provided with treatment, with no significant further deterioration.

Thus, although schizophrenia is, of course, a serious mental illness with sometimes the most severe consequences for the patient and the family, on balance there is more reason to hope for a good to excellent outcome.

While treatment (preferably early) from mental health professionals seems to considerably improve the chances of recovery, there is also evidence that natural processes, which we do not quite understand, lead to eventual stabilization and, in some cases, complete recovery.

## International differences

Over the years, a number of studies of the long-term outcomes of people with schizophrenia have been conducted in countries across the world. In particular, the WHO has drawn together studies of populations in countries as diverse as China, Hong Kong, India, the USA and various countries in Europe. Although there are considerable similarities in the patterns and variations of the way the disease becomes apparent and how people fare over the long term, one consistent finding is that people in developing countries achieve, over time, better levels of social recovery and symptom reduction. This finding caused surprise among researchers.

There is no obvious single factor that can explain the differences between developed and developing countries. One proposed explanation is that of differing gene patterns. However, perhaps more convincing is the fact that mentally ill people are better looked after in traditional rural communities, where they may be provided with simple but rewarding occupations and may be subject to fewer negative emotions within the family. In the UK, Asian populations appear to have lower relapse and re-admission rates, while those of Afro-Caribbean origin have higher relapse rates. These apparent differences have caused considerable debate within the professional and wider community. There is certainly a clear recognition now that some immigrant communities receive poorer levels of mental health care and therefore achieve poorer outcomes. This problem seems to particularly affect Afro-Caribbean communities. However, as with most things in psychiatry, there are no clear explanations. One thing of which we can be sure, the controversy surrounding racial and cultural differences will continue. It is also true to say that the stigma of mental illness is often accentuated by racism.

## The national picture

### The Schizophrenia Commission

In November 2011 the charity Rethink Mental Illness established the Schizophrenia Commission and asked one of the world's leading psychiatrists, Professor Sir Robin Murray, FRS, of the Institute of Psychiatry, King's College London, to chair the process. The independent commission was made up of 14 experts including psychiatrists, a professor of pharmacy, a social worker, a health journalist, a health economist, a general practitioner, a health service manager, representatives of the charitable and voluntary sector and, importantly, two individuals with a diagnosis of schizophrenia. The final report was named *The Abandoned Illness* (The Schizophrenia Commission 2012). We recommend that you read the full report, which is available online (see the References section) and provides a picture of schizophrenia as it exists within the context of twenty-first century Britain.

In many ways, the report serves as a damning indictment of the way in which we as a society provide care and treatment for those affected by this illness. It is also critical of the care for families and carers, and places emphasis on the impact of the illness on those close to the patient. It calls for a radical overhaul of care and treatment services, as well as addressing a number of important background priorities. We will not provide commentary on the report, which runs to nearly 100 pages, as this would not do justice to direct reading. It has an excellent reference section and if you have a particular interest you can find there the sources of the evidence described in the body of the report.

Associated with the Schizophrenia Commission's report are the two reports discussed next: *Effective Interventions in Schizophrenia* (Andrew *et al.* 2012) and the *Report of the National Audit of Schizophrenia* (Royal College of Psychiatrists 2012).

## The Economics of Schizophrenia

The Schizophrenia Commission asked a number of distinguished health economists at the London School of Economics and the Institute of Psychiatry to provide information on the long-term economic impact of schizophrenia and the costs of delivering services. The commission was particularly interested to examine the evidence regarding the costs of effective interventions and to consider ways in which services could be provided in the most cost-effective way. This is not to say for a moment that the commission intended the team to look just for the cheapest options for care and treatment. Rather, it wanted to know about the possible advantages of providing the best-quality care to those with schizophrenia.

The economists found that schizophrenia costs English society £11.8 billion per year and the public sector £7.2 billion. This amounts to an average cost to society, per person with schizophrenia per year, of £60,000 and to the public sector of £36,000. The report demonstrated that the illness causes considerable economic disadvantage; also that the employment rate for people with schizophrenia has fallen very significantly over time. It is estimated that only 15 per cent of people with schizophrenia are now gainfully employed. The economists also considered education and examined the way in which schizophrenia disrupts education in adolescence and early adulthood. They pointed out that the development of the illness means that young people miss education and training opportunities; in turn, the team found that homelessness as a consequence of schizophrenia was much more common than previously thought. They found that no less than 33 per cent of people with schizophrenia in London and Leicester had been homeless at some time. Of these, one-third had a history of sleeping on the streets. Homelessness obviously leads to having no fixed address and hence being unable to open a bank account or seek work. Homelessness itself has very significant costs to society, in addition to the enormous individual impact.

The authors examined the issue of physical health problems, which are more frequent in people with schizophrenia, and pointed out that people with schizophrenia were much less likely to undergo health screening or to be in receipt of simple (and very cheap) measures such as aspirin as a preventative measure for stroke.

The team identified the over-representation of people with schizophrenia within the criminal justice system and reported that there were 2,000 or so people in prison with schizophrenia and nearly 8,000 with a psychotic illness. The authors asked whether many of those people should have been in prison at all. Indeed, wider experience shows that the crimes for which people with schizophrenia are convicted are often minor, and prison becomes an alternative to decent care in hospital or the community.

One of the most important areas that the report covered was the impact of schizophrenia on the family. It showed that the need to care for a family member with schizophrenia has a huge impact on family members because of the loss of work and the need to provide what, in many cases, is substantial amounts of unpaid care, usually by a female family member.

With regard to interventions for schizophrenia, the authors pointed out that using what appear, on the face of it, to be expensive services such as early intervention teams actually leads to financial savings for society. People who have been provided with early interventions are less likely to be admitted to hospital later on and make less use of services than people who have not been provided with early intervention. Likewise, the team found that placement and support schemes in work, albeit initially expensive, led to a range of economic benefits later on. The results of their studies indicated that the most effective interventions could be seen as having real value for money.

Overall, in times when the cost of everything we do in society is subject to intense scrutiny, mental health services seem for many years to have been the poor relation. Although mental health services are targeted at people who have many needs, there are numerous studies to show that compared with problems such as heart disease, cancer and other physical illnesses, mental health services are grossly underfunded. In order to prevent further cuts to mental health budgets and to ensure that mental health services receive more equitable funding, it is essential that the results of this report are taken on board by government. People with schizophrenia and their families need to lobby their local MPs for more support, and the report of the economic analysis conducted by this team of highly regarded international experts should prove to be great ammunition.

## The National Audit of Schizophrenia

In 2012, this audit was the first attempt to develop a comprehensive picture of the quality of care that people with schizophrenia receive in England and Wales. The Royal College of Psychiatrists audited the services provided in 64 NHS mental health trusts in England and Wales. The audit examined a sample of 100 adults with schizophrenia in each of the trusts under study.

The results showed both positive and negative outcomes. While overall there was a level of satisfaction reported by people with schizophrenia and their families, there were clearly major deficits in the services provided. The audit noted that the most serious deficit was in the monitoring and management of physical health problems, stating that the monitoring of risks for cardiovascular illness, which is much more prevalent in people with schizophrenia than the general population, was 'extremely poor'. We have therefore provided in this book substantial information and advice about physical health and illness.

The audit also showed that people with schizophrenia felt they were not sufficiently provided with information about their medication and were not sufficiently involved in the decision about which medication they should take. It found wide variation in the availability of psychological treatments across England and Wales and that one-third of people with schizophrenia had not been offered any form of therapy. The lengthy report of the audit, which amounts to more than 150 pages, is in our opinion required reading for those who want to know more about how services are being provided. Hopefully, the results of this audit will make many trusts think again about the quality of care they provide.

# Part 2
# TREATMENT

# 4

# Introduction to treatment

In this section we will describe the recommended treatments for schizophrenia. Many have been offered in the past, and if you look on the Internet today you will find a multitude of treatment suggestions. We emphasize that in this book we describe only those treatments that have an evidence base and have been tested within rigorous scientific trials.

We believe that treatments for mental health problems are no different from treatments for physical illnesses, although we appreciate that measuring outcomes (whether a treatment improves signs and symptoms) is more difficult than, for example, with cancer. Nevertheless, research methods in mental health have improved and research has become more rigorous in identifying reliable measures of outcome. Thus, any reasonable mental health researcher will say that it is important to measure not just signs and symptoms but also changes in quality of life, satisfaction with treatment, and economic factors such as employment. Our main point of reference for evidence to support a treatment is the National Institute for Health and Care Excellence.

## The National Institute for Health and Care Excellence (NICE)

NICE is an independent organization set up by government to provide national guidance on promoting good health and preventing ill health. It has several functions, one of them being the production of clinical guidelines – evidence-based treatment recommendations. NICE guidelines are published in various forms: a lengthy version, which contains all of the background scientific evidence; an executive summary, which is usually between 10 and 30 pages; and summaries written in plain English. NICE has issued guidance on the treatments for schizophrenia, which is subject to regular updating.

In Chapters 7 and 8 we will describe various approaches to the treatment of schizophrenia, some of which use medications and others that are based on different types of intervention. All the treatments we describe have an evidence base to support their use. We will try to provide a comprehensive account but if you want to know more we suggest you look at the NICE website: <www.nice.org.uk>. This is easy to use and full of information not only about schizophrenia but also all the common physical illnesses and mental health problems.

Many readers will also know that NICE is sometimes referred to in the popular press as 'the drugs-rationing body'. We believe this is unfair; some drugs may cost many thousands of pounds yet yield only limited benefits, so NICE makes recommendations about what drugs can be made available cost-effectively within the limits of NHS resources. Even if the resources of the NHS were to be doubled tomorrow, someone would still have to make recommendations about what we, as a country, can and cannot afford. You may also be interested to know that NICE is the body that regulates medical devices and ensures that they are of the highest standard.

## Treatment choices

Schizophrenia is a condition that requires a combination of medical, psychological, social and spiritual care. Lifestyle choices such as diet, exercise and use of tobacco, alcohol and illicit drugs also can also help or hinder mental health, as we discuss in Chapter 14.

It is more helpful if information about treatment is per-sonalized – specific and tailored to you. When you discuss your treatment choices with health professionals they will take into account things such as gender, age, culture, ethnicity, beliefs, and length and experience of mental health problems. Good mental health care should be a collaborative endeavour between you, your family, friends, health professionals and the wider community. You and your family should be central to any decision made about your care and treatment. However, for you to be truly involved in the decisions about your care you need to have as much information as possible about the choices that are available to you.

# 5

# Professionals: Who are they and what do they do?

Perhaps because of the fear engendered by the topic of mental illness and also because of sometimes highly inaccurate media portrayals, we believe it is important to set out some information concerning mental health professionals. Certainly, if you have schizophrenia or are a family member or carer for someone with schizophrenia you have a right to know about the mental health professionals involved in care and treatment.

All mental health professionals are regulated by professional bodies and professional councils. All professionals, without exception, have signed up to a code of conduct, which means that they have to not only perform their professional role to the best of their ability but also in accord with clearly set out codes of conduct. The other important matter to bear in mind is that of vocational calling. The vast majority of mental health professionals work in the area because they care about mental health, and although their salaries and conditions of work are quite reasonable, many professionals involved in mental health care could easily have taken jobs in other areas that would have provided them with better remuneration and a less stressful working environment. We know that working in mental health care can be very stressful. However, this stress is counterbalanced by the satisfaction obtained from knowing that you might have made a difference to someone's life.

## Some myths

Sadly, much of the knowledge of mental health professionals possessed by the general public derives from films and works of fiction. Many people have a view of inpatient mental health services derived from the film *One Flew Over the Cuckoo's Nest*, where those with mental illness were treated against their will with methods that led to them becoming helpless and subservient. In the same way, community mental health services are often described in highly derogatory terms in the media. From the outset it needs to be emphasized that people who undergo what is often lengthy education and training to become professionally qualified in mental health care do so because of their basic wish to do what they can to reduce the distress caused by a wide range of mental health problems.

People with mental illness in the UK are protected in a wide variety of ways by UK and European law and it is only in a minority of cases that people are deprived of their liberty. If this extreme step is taken, all professionals know that any restrictions on an individual should be for the shortest time possible and that even when restrictions are applied there is an underlying principle that care and treatment must be provided in the least restrictive fashion.

## Psychiatrists

Psychiatrists are doctors who have obtained a basic medical degree and then undertaken the necessary further experience to obtain full registration with the General Medical Council. This further experience usually means spending at least 12 months in two specialities (not mental health) – for example, general medicine or general surgery. Many will then obtain other experience before deciding on a career in psychiatry. It is quite common for doctors who have eventually qualified as psychiatrists to have spent additional time in specialities such as accident and emergency, gynaecology, paediatrics, cancer care and so on.

Once a doctor decides on a career in psychiatry he or she needs to obtain experience in one of the supervised training programmes that lead to membership of the Royal College of Psychiatrists. These training programmes involve 3 years or more of further training and experience. Doctors will only become members of the Royal College of Psychiatrists following examinations – both written and of their skills. Once a member they can undertake so-called 'higher' training that allows them to obtain further experience and education in a speciality such as maternal mental health, forensic psychiatry or community psychiatry. This higher training, accompanied by further experience, will enable that doctor to apply for a post as a consultant psychiatrist. Consultant psychiatrists are the most senior psychiatric doctors in either a hospital or community team. In summary, to become a consultant psychiatrist means, in general, 10 years or more of education, training and experience following initial qualification as a doctor.

As we describe in Chapter 10, psychiatrists have legal powers. For example, a psychiatrist can recommend the admission to hospital of a person under a section of the Mental Health Act. However, only trained psychiatrists who have been approved by the Secretary of State for Health have such powers. Therefore, patients and the general public should be reassured that the considerable responsibilities of a psychiatrist are only given to those with sufficient qualifications and experience. Each patient of a mental health service will have a consultant psychiatrist who remains ultimately responsible for that person's care and treatment. However, some patients are managed by psychiatrists who have not become consultants; rather they are often referred to as staff grade psychiatrists, specialist registrars or similar. Although they are not consultants they are nevertheless doctors with considerable qualifications and experience in psychiatry and there is no reason to suppose that the standard of care they provide is in any way questionable.

## Mental health nurses

Mental health nurses, like general nurses, nurses for those with learning disabilities or children's nurses, have undertaken a 3-year university-based education and training. All nurses, regardless of their eventual speciality, will receive a foundation period of education and training in a range of core skills such as taking blood pressure, temperature and pulse; medication management and administration; giving injections; and developing nursing care plans. In addition, all nurses in the foundation part of their training will obtain some knowledge of all branches of health care, both in the hospital and in the community.

To qualify as a mental health nurse, students will follow on from their foundation training to obtain experience, skills and knowledge in a range of settings relevant to mental health. These include both hospital and community settings and, within these, experience in specialities such as the mental health care of older people, children and adolescents; forensic psychiatry; assertive outreach teams and so on. When they have passed their university examinations they must register with the Nursing and Midwifery Council. This regulates the activities of all nurses and midwives in the UK and issues a code of conduct that ensures nurses are able to provide their skills and knowledge to the highest possible level. The council remains responsible by law for the conduct of nurses and midwives and is able to remove nurses from the register for misconduct if they fail to meet professional standards.

Once qualified, mental health nurses often receive further education and training. This may include skills in psychological therapies – notably CBT – and many nurses nowadays undertake further education and training at master's degree level. An increasing number of mental health nurses progress even further to undertake a PhD. There are also hundreds of mental health nurses across the country who have obtained research knowledge and skills and work within all of the major research initiatives.

An important development in the last 10 years has been the advent of the nurse prescriber. It has long been recognized that one of the problems of delivering health care in general, and mental health care in particular, has been a shortage of doctors who may prescribe the appropriate medication and then monitor and review the medication in the long term. Some years ago, the UK government put into law the provision for nurses to become prescribers. This prescriptive authority is only conferred once a nurse has received an appropriately comprehensive programme of education and training. Remember that for many years midwives have been able to prescribe powerful painkilling drugs such as pethidine without a doctor's authority. In the USA, nurse prescribing has been a feature of the health care system for some time. All parts of the UK now have nurse prescribers in mental health and many people with schizophrenia will have contact with a one.

Broadly, there are two types of nurse prescriber:

*Supplementary prescribers* can take some responsibility for varying a basic prescription made by a doctor. This may include changing the frequency of a dose, increasing or decreasing a dose and conducting – on the doctor's behalf – reviews of medication.

*Independent prescribers* can, like midwives, prescribe medications without a doctor's authority. In practice this will often mean that they work alongside the medically qualified psychiatrist. Thus, for example, the psychiatrist may prescribe the main antipsychotic medications; however, the independent nurse prescriber may be called upon to prescribe some additional tranquillizing medication or medication to deal with side effects.

It is important to emphasize that once someone with schizophrenia is in the care of mental health services they are always in the care of a team of people, although one person may take the main responsibility for prescribing. Often, it is a mental health nurse who knows the person best and sees them most frequently. It therefore becomes logical for that person to adjust medication or make new prescriptions. Many psychiatrists will often say that not only is the mental health nurse the person who knows the patient best, but many mental health nurses have many years of experience within their speciality. This experience, together with their education and training, makes them highly suitable individuals to take on wider responsibilities for patient care.

## Mental health social workers

As with other professions, social work has undergone considerable developments over the past 50 years. At one time social workers were trained from the outset to work in a particular area – for example, in hospital. In mental health care, some social workers were specifically trained as mental welfare officers.

For many reasons, social work education and training underwent considerable change, and social workers now undertake a general education and training in social work at university. This training involves all aspects of social work, including working with children and families, those in residential care and, of course, people with mental health problems.

Those who wish to specialize in mental health can then obtain further education and training to become 'approved' social workers. This enables them not only to work in mental health care, but also to perform various legal roles and functions within the Mental Health Act and other legislation relevant to people with mental health problems. Social workers are generally employed by local authorities. At one time this caused problems because their employment was separate from that of health professionals, who, one way or another, worked for the NHS. This situation has been resolved to a great extent, and although the pay of social workers comes from a source outside the NHS, mental health social workers are now considered to be part of the mental health team.

Mental health social workers deal with a range of matters (apart from their legal responsibilities), including helping people with schizophrenia navigate their way around the complex benefits system. This has become even more difficult because of recent changes, including tests for availability for work. Social workers can often be very helpful in identifying suitable housing associations that are particularly appropriate for those with mental health problems. Most social workers will also have considerable skills in providing the necessary emotional support to families and, when children are involved in the family structure, they will be able to provide the right advice and help.

## Occupational therapists

Like their nursing and social work colleagues, occupational therapists undertake general training in their core profession before specializing in mental health. They have great expertise in helping people with the activities of daily living. In hospital settings, occupational therapists are central to the organization and planning of the patient's day. They are responsible for setting up and providing various groups and activities, ranging from relaxation and exercise programmes to activities that provide helpful diversion, such as the traditional creative activities such as pottery and art. Some have a particular interest in using art or drama as a vehicle for therapy and may have undertaken further education and training in these areas.

Occupational therapists also work within community mental health teams and have particular skills in rehabilitation. Thus, people recovering from an acute episode of illness will benefit from the skilled advice and support that the occupational therapist can provide. They help the person to regain a normal routine, help with the development of job interview skills and identify employment possibilities. For those who are about to live independently for the first time, occupational therapists can help them adjust to the day-to-day activities that most of us have to face, such as shopping, laundry and housework.

Apart from these practical matters, occupational therapists have particular expertise in the assessment of the individual's function. By a process of observation and the completion of assessment tools they are able to provide their colleagues in the mental health team with valuable information to assist with the overall process of care, treatment and rehabilitation.

Occupational therapists are regulated by the Health and Care Professions Council and in the same way as doctors and nurses need to adhere to a code of conduct and demonstrate that they keep their skills and knowledge up to date.

## Psychologists

The psychologists employed by mental health services will, in general, be clinical psychologists. However, there are other psychologists whose qualifications, background and experience are somewhat different.

All psychologists have undertaken an undergraduate degree in psychology. The undergraduate degree covers a wide range of topics, including an understanding of behaviour, learning, memory and social interaction. In addition, a degree in psychology also includes the acquisition of knowledge and skills in conducting research, such as the use of statistical analysis and experimental methodology.

After their first degree, those who wish to pursue a career in clinical psychology will often obtain further experience working as an assistant in a research programme or for a qualified clinical psychologist in a hospital or community setting. Once they have obtained the relevant experience they embark on a further 3 years of university-based education and training that leads them to qualify as a clinical psychologist. Today, most clinical psychologist qualifications will confer the title 'doctor', although clinical psychologists who qualified some years ago will not have this title.

The training programme for clinical psychology will include experience in a wide range of areas relevant to mental health and may also include experience in other settings, such as learning disabilities and general hospitals. Once a clinical psychologist has qualified, he or she – like their psychiatric colleagues – will undertake further education, training and periods of experience before reaching the most senior levels.

Much of the work of clinical psychologists in mental health services today involves providing psychological therapies, principally CBT. However, clinical psychologists are also responsible for the supervision of others who provide psychological therapy. Clinical psychologists also have important roles in respect of the assessment of patients. They may undertake highly specialized testing of thinking and memory, and some clinical psychologists will also have skills in neuropsychology and thus be able to assess and provide treatment to people who have had a brain injury.

The clinical psychologist will, in partnership with other team members, be responsible for designing programmes of rehabilitation, and their specialist knowledge of memory and learning will be of great assistance in setting treatment targets.

As we have mentioned, clinical psychologists are not the only psychologists in mental health services. There is now the speciality of health psychology. Health psychologists have received specific training in a number of areas relevant to the issue of general health and psychological function. Some examples of the work that health psychologists undertake are to be found in the provision of the psychological support that is so necessary in cardiac rehabilitation, weight loss programmes and adherence to medical treatments, including medication. Health psychologists can also assist with interventions for one of the most important problems that affects people with schizophrenia, that of tobacco addiction.

All psychologists employed within mental health services are regulated by the Health and Care Professions Council and are usually members of the British Psychological Society, the professional body for psychology in the UK.

## Cognitive behavioural therapists

In recent times there has been recognition that there have been insufficient numbers of professionals who are skilled in CBT. To rectify this the government has set up a programme entitled 'Improving Access to Psychological Therapies'. This programme has involved recruiting people from professional and non-professional backgrounds to train as cognitive behavioural therapists. Some of these individuals are now employed within mental health services and in general are to be found in community settings. CBT is an important intervention in schizophrenia (see Chapter 8). However, as the National Audit found (see Chapter 3), there is wide variation in the availability of psychological treatments across the countries of the UK. Sadly, only one-third of people with schizophrenia had been offered any form of therapy. Thus the recent initiative to train more cognitive behavioural therapists is most welcome.

## Support workers

Community mental health teams employ support workers. These are equivalent to the nursing assistants and health care assistants in general hospital settings. Support workers do as their name suggests – they provide support to professionals, who may delegate various therapy tasks to them, and they also support people with schizophrenia within their care and treatment programmes. Support workers may therefore assist with activities of daily living, helping the person in respect of a range of tasks – everything from going to the gym to doing the weekly shop. They will also help those who are very disabled by their illness by providing practical assistance with the basic activities of daily living.

## General practitioners and primary health care

In many books and guidelines concerning schizophrenia, the role of the GP and the primary health care team is often missing. In our opinion, the GP is an important figure in the professional treatment of schizophrenia. It is more likely than not that the health professional who knows the patient best will be their own GP. Indeed, the GP may be the first person to be called upon to make an assessment of a patient's mental state.

At one time, many GPs had little or no knowledge of the assessment and treatment of mental health problems. However, this situation is changing rapidly. To become a fully qualified GP, doctors need to undertake specialist training in general practice over a 3-year period. Many doctors will include a 6-month training period in a mental health service and will obtain knowledge and skills over and above those they obtained in their first medical degree. Many GPs thus have quite reasonable knowledge of schizophrenia. In addition to specialist mental health experience, some GPs will have undertaken further education and training in mental health topics. However, it is also true to say that, although these advances in the training and education of doctors are to be welcomed, there are still many GPs who have poor levels of knowledge and skills about not only schizophrenia but also a wide range of mental health topics. In addition, many GPs will tell you that the amount of time they can allocate to each patient is limited and this shortage of time compromises their ability to properly understand the individual.

Once the diagnosis of schizophrenia is established it is vital that the patient maintains reasonable contact with the GP, in addition to contact with other mental health professionals. The GP should remain central to the provision of health care and, given that people with schizophrenia are more susceptible than the general population to a range of physical health problems, it is important that they attend their GP surgery for health screening (see Chapter 13), including blood pressure monitoring, testing of cholesterol and blood sugar levels and screening for breast, cervical and testicular cancers.

# 6

# Where should treatment and care take place?

Fifty years or so ago, most people who received a diagnosis of schizophrenia were treated in hospital. In the 1950s there were something in the order of 160,000 beds in large mental hospitals in the UK, which were typically set in the countryside surrounding big cities. Many of these hospitals were built in the Victorian era and it was common to find some hospitals with more than 2,000 beds and wards containing 50 or more patients. These hospitals were autonomous communities, often containing a farm that provided produce for the hospital kitchens and offering a range of services such as upholstery departments and large laundries. Patients were often sent to work in these facilities as part of their treatment, although following the Second World War many of the large hospitals began to offer various psychological and rehabilitation therapies. These were to become more common, particularly during the 1960s and 1970s.

The 1959 Mental Health Act emphasized the need for people to be admitted voluntarily, where possible, as informal patients rather than confined under legal orders or 'sections'. The 1959 Act enshrined the principle of providing care in the least restrictive fashion – a principle also underpinning current legislation (the 1983 Mental Health Act, which has subsequently been subject to various revisions).

It may come as a surprise to some to know that Enoch Powell, a politician known for his extreme views on immigration, was one of those who argued for the closure of mental hospitals and their replacement with facilities in the community. He made his famous 'water tower' speech in 1961. Powell, then the Minister of Health, argued for 'the elimination of by far the greater part of this country's mental hospitals as they exist today'. He went on to say:

> This is a colossal undertaking, not so much in the new physical provision which it involves, as in the sheer inertia of mind and matter which it requires to be overcome. There they stand, isolated,

majestic, imperious, brooded over by the gigantic water tower and chimney combined, rising unmistakable and daunting out of the countryside – the asylums which our forefathers built with such immense solidity to express the notions of their day. Do not for a moment underestimate their powers of resistance to our assault.

Just months after this, US President Kennedy was announcing the opening of community mental health centres and the closure of a large number of state asylums.

Over the years the number of beds available for inpatient care in the UK has fallen from 160,000 to something in the order of 20,000, and the large mental hospitals in England and Wales have closed. Some of them were turned into housing estates and others retained their listed building status and ironically offer accommodation in expensive apartments. Elsewhere, large supermarkets occupy the land where mental hospitals once stood. This sale has been a bone of contention for advocates of increased funding for mental health services as it yielded great financial returns but the proceeds were not returned to the funding of modern mental health services and instead were returned to the Exchequer for general use.

## Community treatment

For the past 40 years or so there has been a considerable emphasis on providing, where possible, care and treatment in the community. There is a wide range of research that shows that people with schizophrenia and their families prefer care and treatment to take place at home. Other research shows that community services produce much better outcomes in respect of symptoms, daily functioning and quality of life. A history of how community services developed is interesting but out of place here, so if you would like to read further take a look at Thornicroft *et al.* (2011) for a more detailed account.

There remains wide (although not 100 per cent) agreement among mental health professionals that we still need to provide inpatient care for those whose illness is severe and who require 24-hour skilled medical and nursing care. Unfortunately, in the depth of an acute episode of schizophrenia, some people are unable to see that they require care and treatment and then it becomes necessary to use legal powers under the 1983 Mental Health Act to compulsorily admit and detain them in hospital.

## The Care Programme Approach

The Care Programme Approach is of central importance for those with mental health problems. It was set up by government more than two decades ago to ensure that people with more serious mental health problems did not slip through the net of care. Prior to this it was common to see people with illnesses such as schizophrenia passing through the NHS without anyone being made to take responsibility for their care and treatment. As most readers will know, some people with schizophrenia can at times be so disabled by their condition that they are unable to access the help they need. In the past this situation has led to high-profile tragedies. Although these still occur, they occur much less frequently than before. You will find a great deal of information about the Care Programme Approach on the NHS website <http://www.nhs.uk/CarersDirect/guide/mental-health/Pages/care-programme-approach.aspx>.

The Care Programme Approach makes the NHS responsible for providing an assessment of anyone with a significant mental health problem by a qualified mental health professional. That professional is responsible for identifying the nature of the person's illness and their treatment and care needs. The approach also requires the professional to identify the carers of those with mental illness and to assess them also for their needs for support. The person with the illness should be allocated a care coordinator, commonly a community mental health nurse, social worker or other mental health professional. Health services generally try to nominate a care coordinator who has a good relationship with the person and who will remain for an indefinite period.

The approach applies equally to people in hospital and in the community. Treatment is governed by a care plan, which identifies areas of need, any risks, and plans in case of an emergency or crisis. The person who is subject to the Care Programme Approach will be provided with contact details should an emergency or crisis arise and there is an obligation for the NHS to provide 24-hour access 7 days a week for all those in need. The care plans are reviewed when anything changes in the person's situation and in any case at intervals of usually 6 months.

# 7

# Medication

Before you make a decision about medication it is likely you will want to know more about the choice of medicines available to you, how they work, how effective they are likely to be, what side effects they might cause, what you can do to minimize and manage side effects and how long you will need to take it for.

A range of medicines are used to treat schizophrenia, including antipsychotics, antidepressants and mood stabilizers. The most commonly used medications – antipsychotics – have been available to treat schizophrenia since the 1950s. The earlier drugs are known as either 'conventional', 'typical' or 'first-generation' antipsychotics; these drugs include chlorpromazine and haloperidol. The more recent drugs are known as 'atypical' or 'second-generation' antipsychotics and include clozapine, risperidone, olanzapine, quetiapine and amisulpride. 'Third-generation' antipsychotics include aripiprazole.

These medicines can be taken in tablet or liquid form and need to be taken one or twice a day. Most of them also come in a short-acting or long-acting injectable form. The short-acting injections are usually given in emergency situations when someone is very distressed and would like to be or needs to be calmed quickly. Long-acting injections (also known as 'depot' injections) need only be given once every 2–4 weeks. Injections, whether they are short acting or long acting are given into the muscle. When having regular injections, alternating injection sites is important to prevent pain and physical health problems such as abscesses. There are a number of sites on the body where an injection can be administered. The most common site is the upper part of the bottom (the dorsogluteal site), though there are four other suitable places – just below the hip (the ventrogluteal site), the outer thigh (the vastus lateralis muscle) and the top of the arm (the deltoid muscle), although risperidone and paliperidone are the only antipsychotics that can be currently administered in the deltoid muscle.

How to take medication should be a joint decision between you and your prescriber. If you are unhappy with how you take your medication it is important to discuss this with your mental health team so that your experience can be improved.

All medicines for physical and mental health conditions have at least two names: a generic name (e.g. clozapine), which is the active ingredient of the drug, and a brand name given by the manufacturer (e.g. Clozaril or Zaponex). When a pharmaceutical company discovers a new drug it files for a patent, which lasts about 20 years. No other company can make the drug while it is protected under patent. However, once the patent expires any company can manufacture a 'generic' version and sell it under a new brand name. Before a generic drug is sold it has to pass

**Table 2 Commonly used antipsychotic medicines**

| Generic name | Brand name | Formulation |
| --- | --- | --- |
| Amisulpride | Solian | Tablet and liquid |
| Aripiprazole | Abilify | Tablet, liquid, dispersible tablet, short-acting injection |
| Chlorpromazine | Largactil, Thorazine | Tablet, liquid, short-acting injection |
| Clozapine | Clozaril, Zaponex, Denzapine | Tablet and liquid |
| Flupentixol | Depixol, Fluanxol | Tablet and long-acting injection |
| Fluphenazine | Modecate, Prolixin | Tablet and long-acting injection |
| Haloperidol | Haldol | Tablet, liquid, short- and long-acting injections |
| Olanzapine | Zyprexa, Zypadhera | Tablet, dispersible tablet, short- and long-acting injections |
| Paliperidone | Invega, Xeplion | Tablet and long-acting injection |
| Quetiapine | Seroquel | Tablet |
| Risperidone | Risperdal | Tablet, liquid, dispersible tablet, long-acting injection |
| Zuclopenthixol | Clopixol | Tablet, short- and long-acting injections |

strict tests to ensure that it is not different from the original product; for example, the dose has to be the same as well as the way it works on the body. The shape, colour and taste of the drug are likely to change, however. The biggest difference is cost. The new version made by a different company is much cheaper than the original drug (e.g. Zaponex is considerably cheaper than Clozaril). It is cheaper because the research, development and marketing costs of the drug have already been paid for by the company that developed it. Hospital pharmacies will often buy the new version to save money. To avoid any unnecessary confusion, the person who is prescribing your medicine or the pharmacy who dispenses it should tell you if they are going to give you an alternative (and cheaper) version of your medicine. The new drug will work in exactly the same way but it may look and taste different.

Table 2 contains a list of commonly used antipsychotic medicines and the different ways you can take them.

## How long will they take to work?

In recent years, clinicians have found that if a particular anti-psychotic drug is going to work, most improvement is likely to be seen in the first 2 weeks – providing it is taken as prescribed at a therapeutic dose. If there is no change in symptoms at all then a switch to another drug is recommended after 2–3 weeks. This does not mean you should stop taking the medicine after 2 weeks if you start to feel better. For antipsychotics to have the best effect they need to be taken long term as they will continue to help your mental health improve.

## How effective are antipsychotics?

Antipsychotics provide control over symptoms. According to a number of research studies (Leucht *et al.* 2009), clozapine is the most effective antipsychotic for treating overall symptoms. Olanzapine, risperidone and amisulpride are all equally effective but not as effective as clozapine in treating symptoms. Quetiapine, aripiprazole and haloperidol are more or less equally effective but not as effective as the other antipsychotics. For depressive symptoms within the context of schizophrenia, quetiapine and aripiprazole seem to be as effective as the other antipsychotics.

Antipsychotic medication will be effective in approximately 8 out of 10 people. It is important to understand what clinicians mean when they talk about a medicine being 'effective'. It usually means a reduction in symptoms, not that the symptoms will completely disappear, and you can usually expect at least a 50 per cent reduction in symptoms. For those whose symptoms do not respond sufficiently to olanzapine, risperidone or amisulpride, then clozapine is likely to effective in about 60–70 per cent of people. For a small group of people symptoms will completely disappear but another small group of people may still experience distressing symptoms despite an optimal amount of medication. If you ask people who are prescribed medication what they find helpful about it, they will usually say they are not as bothered by their voices or experiences, which somehow fade into the background, and it helps them cope.

Taking medication is only one part of staying well, albeit an important part – psychological interventions are needed to help people make sense of their experiences (see Chapter 8). Taking your medication regularly will not absolutely guarantee that you will stay well; however, it greatly increases your chances of staying well. In a group of ten people with schizophrenia, all taking their medication regularly, one of them, on average, will relapse within a year and the other nine, providing they were well supported in other areas of their lives, are likely to remain well. In another group of ten people who stop taking their medication too early in their recovery, about 70 per cent will relapse with a year. Long-term mental health is much better in people who have fewer relapses or when relapses are of a short duration.

## How does antipsychotic medication work and why does it cause side effects?

Antipsychotics work by increasing or reducing the effects of natural chemicals (neurotransmitters) in the brain, including dopamine, serotonin, noradrenaline and acetylcholine. These neurotransmitters control various aspects of our behaviour, including mood and emotions, sleeping, wakefulness and eating. A feature shared by all antipsychotic medicines is their ability to reduce the amount of dopamine in the brain by blocking dopamine receptors. One the one hand this is useful because, as we discussed in Chapter 2, too much dopamine in a particular part of the brain may be related to experiences such as voices and paranoid thinking, so blocking its effects may help to dampen their importance and significance. However, although there have been advances in the design of new medicines in the last 20 years, antipsychotic drugs are still not that sophisticated and some (but not all) block dopamine receptors and other types of receptors in the brain that lead to unwanted effects (side effects).

For example, some of the older medicines such as chlorpromazine and haloperidol also block dopamine in a part of the brain where there is not enough. This is unhelpful, as reducing dopamine even further in this part of the brain is likely to make some experiences worse; for example, not having any interest and motivation to do things or finding it difficult to make conversation. Some drugs also affect dopamine receptors in two other pathways in the brain and are the cause of additional unpleasant effects. Movement disorders such as shaking hands, 'restless legs' and abnormal facial move- ments are caused by blocking dopamine in the part of the brain that controls how we move. Sexual problems such as lack of interest in sex, poor sexual performance, lack of satisfaction, painful, swollen breasts (in both men and women) and periods stopping are caused by blocking dopamine neurotransmission in the part of the brain that controls the regulation of a hormone called prolactin. Sexual side effects are not only caused by altering (i.e. raising) the levels of prolactin, they can be caused by the effect of the medicine on other parts of the brain and body. Some antipsychotic medicines (the older and newer ones) block additional receptors in the brain, such as histamine receptors. Blocking a particular type of hista- mine receptor may cause you to feel tired and lethargic and to gain weight. Low blood pressure, dizziness, dry mouth, constipation and blurred vision are all caused by the medicine's effect on different types of receptors in the brain.

Side effects are related to the dose and frequency of a medicine, also how long a drug stays in the body before it is excreted and the health of other parts of the body such as the stomach, liver and kidneys. To get the best out of your medicine you should

**Table 3 Antipsychotics and related side effects**

| Symptom | Amisulpride | Aripiprazole | Chlorpromazine | Clozapine | Haloperidol | Olanzapine | Paliperiaone | Quetiapine | Risperidone |
|---|---|---|---|---|---|---|---|---|---|
| Drowsiness | ✗ | ✗ | ✓✓✓ | ✓✓✓ | ✓ | ✓✓ | ✓ | ✓✓ | ✓ |
| Trembling, muscle spasms | ✓ | ✓/✗ | ✓✓ | ✗ | ✓✓✓ | ✓/✗ | ✓ | ✗ | ✓ |
| Weight gain | ✓ | ✓/✗ | ✓✓ | ✓✓✓ | ✓ | ✓✓✓ | ✓✓ | ✓✓ | ✓✓ |
| Dry mouth, constipation | ✗ | ✗ | ✓✓ | ✓✓✓ | ✓ | ✓ | ✓ | ✓ | ✓ |
| Low blood pressure | ✗ | ✗ | ✓✓✓ | ✓✓✓ | ✓ | ✓ | ✓✓ | ✓✓ | ✓✓ |
| Diabetes | ✓ | ✗ | ✓✓ | ✓✓✓ | ✓/✗ | ✓✓✓ | ✓ | ✓✓ | ✓ |
| Sexual side effects (from high prolactin levels) | ✓✓✓ | ✗ | ✓✓✓ | ✗ | ✓✓✓ | ✓ | ✓✓✓ | ✗ | ✓✓✓ |

Incidence/severity: ✓✓✓ = high; ✓✓ = moderate; ✓ = low; ✓/✗ low to very low, ✗ = very low.

Adapted from *The Maudsley Prescribing Guidelines in Psychiatry* (Taylor et al. 2012).

take the right dose at the right time. This ensures that you always have a stable level in your blood. Side effects can also be kept to a minimum by taking into account factors such as age, gender and the length of time symptoms have been present. For example, a young woman with her first experience of symptoms needs a smaller dose than a man who has been ill for a number of years. A high intake of alcohol over a long period of time can affect the health and function of the liver and kidneys and it may take longer to metabolize a drug; a smaller dose of a medicine will therefore be needed than for someone who is physically healthy.

The person who prescribes your medication and the health care professionals who are part of your care team should be aware of which medicines work on which receptors and should tell you about the good things and not so good things about the medicine you choose. All medicines have side effects, whether they are for the treatment of high blood pressure, diabetes, an infection or a mental health condition. We know which drugs cause which side effects; however, what we do not know for sure is which people will experience a particular side effect and which people will be fortunate enough to avoid it. Research is currently being undertaken on how best to tailor a particular medicine to each individual patient, so as to increase its efficacy but avoid causing side effects. This type of personalized medicine is a few years away from being accessible to everyone. In the meantime, if you are fully aware of which drugs work best and which cause a particular side effect then you are in a better position to participate in decisions about your treatment.

Table 3 is a guide to commonly used antipsychotic medicines and the side effects you might expect. You need to remember that everyone is different and some people may be sensitive to a particular medicine and have a side effect that is uncommon for a particular drug, whereas other people will be more resilient and might avoid experiencing a common side effect associated with a particular drug.

## Managing side effects

Sometimes it can be a delicate balance between achieving relief from distressing symptoms and avoiding side effects. Prevention, early identification, and implementation of management strategies can minimize side effects and improve the experience of taking

**Table 4 Management strategies for the side effects of antipsychotic medication**

| Symptom | Management |
| --- | --- |
| Drowsiness | This usually wears off after a few weeks and can actually be useful in the first few weeks of treatment to help you feel rested. However, if it persists talk to your prescriber about taking your medicine in divided doses throughout the day – smaller doses in the morning and most of it before bedtime. If you no longer need a drug that is sedating then ask for a change in medication. |
| Movement disorders such as trembling or muscles spasms | These are best treated by reducing the dose or switching to a different medication. You can take an additional medication to treat any shakiness or muscle spasms but this is not recommended in the long term. No one should have to tolerate antipsychotic-induced movement disorders as there are plenty of other choices of medicines available that cause little or no movement disorders (see Table 3). |
| Weight gain | As with any medicine you take, it is helpful for you and your care team to take a proactive approach to prevent weight gain. You should weigh yourself regularly and measure your waist circumference. Take into account that your appetite may be much stronger and you might crave foods that relieve hunger quickly, such as chocolate, sweets, cakes, fizzy drinks and fast food. Try to plan ahead, learn how to read food labels and how to make healthy snacks and meals. Most mental health services have exercise instructors and dieticians who can support you in safely increasing your level of activity and eating healthily. Alternatively, you might be able to get a discount at your local gym with the help of your care coordinator. It takes effort to keep your weight stable when on some medicines. If you are unhappy with the effects of your medicine on your weight speak to your prescriber and ask for an alternative. |

| Symptom | Management |
| --- | --- |
| Dry mouth, constipation and blurred vision | A high-fibre diet that includes plenty of fruit and vegetables is helpful. Drink water rather than fizzy drinks, and sugar-free gum for a dry mouth might help. It is important to look after your oral hygiene: it helps to brush your teeth twice a day and have regular dental checkups, as a dry mouth can lead to tooth pain and loss. |
| Low blood pressure (dizziness, feeling faint and light-headed) | Have your blood pressure taken regularly, make sure you are not dehydrated and avoid alcohol, heavy meals, prolonged periods of lying down, long periods of standing still and very hot baths and showers. If it persists discuss with your prescriber the possibility of switching to a drug that does not cause low blood pressure. |
| Raised blood sugar, diabetes | As with weight gain, a proactive approach is needed to prevent changes in blood sugar and the onset of diabetes. The level of glucose in your blood should be tested before a medicine is prescribed, then every 3 months and, when stable, every 6 months. A healthy lifestyle – a good diet, keeping active and not smoking – helps to maintain stable blood sugar levels. Report symptoms such as frequently passing water, increased thirst and abdominal pain to your care coordinator. |
| Sexual side effects (from high prolactin levels) | Report any changes in your interest, performance and satisfaction with sex, as well as swollen, leaking breasts (in both men and women) and erratic periods. Discuss with your prescriber either reducing the dose or switching to a drug that does not cause these side effects. Make sure you follow health promotion advice, e.g. breast self-examination and contraceptive advice. |

medication. Your prescriber or care coordinator should regularly review side effects with a standardized rating scale. Table 4 contains suggestions for managing common side effects.

## How long will I need to take medication for?

This is a decision that only you and your doctor can make (with input from your family). Early and consistent treatment can lead to better outcomes in the future, such as staying out of hospital, getting a job and having good relationships with others. This is not unique to people with schizophrenia. We know that people with other long-term conditions such as depression, diabetes and asthma respond much better to early and consistent treatment than those who wait many years to be treated or go for long periods without medication.

When medication starts working and you feel better it can be tempting to stop taking it. Like people with diabetes, high blood pressure and asthma, many people with mental illness will need to take medication on an ongoing basis to prevent their symptoms coming back. Usually you need to take medication for at least a year or two after recovering from a first episode. If you have a second episode you will need to take medication for up to 5 years before your doctor reviews the treatment. It is very important to talk with your doctor before reducing or stopping any medication.

## What will happen if I stop taking medication?

The decision whether or not to take medicine ultimately lies with you. There are times when you may be in hospital receiving treatment under the Mental Health Act and your freedom to make decisions about your medication is restricted. Even so, the hospital team should make every effort to make you feel involved in the decisions made about your care.

Approximately 50 per cent of people who are prescribed medication stop taking it within a year, and against medical advice. This is not unique to people with schizophrenia. This happens in every health condition for which long-term medication is needed, for a number of reasons. For example, people think they are no longer ill and therefore do not need the drugs, the side effects may be intolerable or they are worried about the long-term effects.

## How to improve the experience of taking medication

We know for certain that if medication is prescribed in a skilled way and you continue to take it regularly you have a much better chance of staying out of hospital. Staying well and out of hospital is obviously important; however, being able to experience a good quality of life whereby you can socialize, have meaningful relation-ships, live independently and work is also vital. These factors need to be taken into account when choosing medication. If you are wanting to prioritize maintaining a job and need to be out of the house for 8.00 a.m. then a medicine that makes you feel tired in the morning may not be the best choice, In turn, for someone in a relationship and where a satisfying sex life is important, medication that causes sexual dysfunction will be unhelpful, to say the least.

Medication can help you achieve the things you want in life, but if it is prescribed badly and side effects are not prevented or minimized you may become discouraged and want to stop it. Improving the experience of taking antipsychotic medica-tion needs a joint effort between you and your family, mental health team and GP. The prescribing and taking of medication is a dynamic and ongoing process. Each management plan needs to be tailored to you and your expectations and managed in a realistic and transparent way.

Meetings between clients, carers and health professionals are time limited. To make the best use of this time you may find it helpful to prepare a list of questions beforehand. It can also help you feel more involved in the decisions made about your care. Here is a list of questions you might like to ask the doctor or nurse pre-scribing your medication:

What choice of medication is available to me?
How does it work?
How effective is it?
Which of my symptoms will it help?
Which of my symptoms will it not help?
What are the side effects associated with this medication?
What is the best way to manage the side effects?
How long will I have to take the medication?
What will happen if/when I stop it?
Do I need any special blood tests/health checks while I am taking it?
Do I have to avoid certain food or drink if I take this medication?
How often will the medication be reviewed?
If I choose not to take medication what other choices are available to me?

When you are taking the medication you should expect your prescriber and mental health team to:

- involve you in any decision made about medication, such as the choice, dose and frequency;
- prescribe the lowest effective dose of the medication once your symptoms are stabilized;
- ideally prescribe a single antipsychotic, rather than more than one, except when you are switching medicines;
- regularly monitor your response to the medication and respond to any new side effects;
- assess your physical health before you start medication and on a regular basis; blood tests and other physical tests such as blood pressure and weight measurement should be part of routine care;
- listen to your views and those of your family if you want to change or stop medication and work with you towards a collaborative agreement.

## Negotiating coming off medication

If you want to stop taking your medication, it is a really important to discuss this with your family, the person who prescribes your medication and the rest of your care team. Some people will have had a positive experience of discussing coming off medication with their health care professionals, while others may have felt not listened to or misunderstood. One reason health professionals can be negative about coming off medication is that many of them come into contact with only the most ill people, as these are the people who are more likely to use specialist mental health services. People who remain well are usually cared for by their family doctor or receive support from voluntary or independent organizations and may never come into contact with mental health services. This means mental health professionals often do not get feedback from clients who improve; they do not see mentally healthy, well-functioning people. They may thus be pessimistic about the potential for recovery and be overly cautious, thinking that everyone should stay on medication for fear of relapse, as they only see people who relapse and have to deal with the sometimes devastating consequences.

We know that stopping antipsychotic medication abruptly doubles the risk of relapse compared with gradual withdrawal. However, little research or advice exists to guide health professionals in supporting clients coming off or reducing medication, and this rarely happens in a planned and systematic way. The box lists the factors your prescriber should consider when you ask to stop or reduce your medication.

When stopping long-term oral and depot antipsychotic medication, the prescriber should carry out a risk–benefit analysis of the client's medication. This should include:

- Current symptoms; if no symptoms are present, what is the length of time the client has been symptom free (long-standing symptoms that are not distressing and have previously been unresponsive to medication may be excluded)?
- Frequency and severity of side effects.
- Previous pattern of illness (speed of onset, duration and severity of episode, danger to self and others).
- Current social circumstances – is the client stable or do they have anticipated life stressors?
- Social cost of a relapse to the client (e.g. sole breadwinner, impact on children).
- Is the client able to monitor their symptoms; if so will they seek help?
- If the client is on oral medication and a depot (long-acting formulation), oral medications should be discontinued first.
- Intervals between injections should be increased to up to 4 weeks before decreasing the dose each time (different rules will apply to risperidone and olanzapine long-acting injections).
- The dose should be reduced by less than one-third at a time.
- Reductions should be made no more frequently than every 3 months (preferably every 6 months).
- If the client becomes symptomatic as a result of the planned withdrawal of medication this should not be seen as failure but rather as an important step in determining the minimum effective dose that the client requires.

Adapted from *The Maudsley Prescribing Guidelines in Psychiatry* (Taylor *et al.* 2012).

# 8

# Non-medical therapies

## Cognitive behavioural therapy

Although people with schizophrenia are entitled to treatment from a mental health professional, CBT, which is recommended in the NICE guidelines, can be applied very effectively as a self-help method. We recommend an excellent book, *Cognitive Behaviour Therapy for Dummies*, by Rhena Branch and Rob Willson. Another useful book, often used by professionals, is *Cognitive Behavioural Therapy Explained*, by Graeme Whitfield and Allan Davidson. It is presented in a readable format and covers therapies for a wide range of problems, including schizophrenia.

CBT has been developed over the last 60 years, first to treat conditions such as phobias, depression and general anxiety. In the last 20 years or so it has been used with considerable success by people with schizophrenia. In our opinion it is essential that all people with schizophrenia are at least assessed for their suitability for CBT and, in the case of people who suffer from the distress of hallucinations or exhibit delusional thinking, CBT should be considered to be as important as medication. While there is a great deal that people with schizophrenia can do for themselves, and that their families can do, in our view it is important that a person with schizophrenia is assisted to use cognitive behavioural methods by a practitioner who has received the appropriate training. In the NHS, clinical psychologists, nurses and an increasing number of other professionals have been provided with CBT training, such as occupational therapists, social workers and therapists within the 'Improving Access to Psychological Therapies' programme.

In CBT, the therapist works actively with the person in the spirit of collaboration so as to identify thoughts, feelings, attitudes and behaviours that may need modification. The initial assessment process involves the therapist simply getting to know the person and obtaining information about their background, family, upbringing, schooling and so on, with a strong focus on getting to know the person as an individual. The person's problems will also be assessed, identifying those that give rise to particular distress or problems with daily living. The therapist will want to know about behaviours and, in particular, unhelpful behaviours such as avoidance or an inability to engage in the usual activities of daily living. The assessment process is also particularly helpful in identifying the person's strengths. As we see in the case study of Sarah, later in the chapter, the focus on the person's strengths may be an important part of therapy.

CBT is a treatment that attempts to change unhelpful thoughts, beliefs, attitudes and behaviours – particularly important in the case of someone with schizophrenia. At assessment it is important to obtain a detailed perspective of particular thoughts and beliefs that give rise to problems. Thus, the client may be asked to keep a diary or fill in questionnaires, which provide the therapist with helpful information.

By the end of the assessment process, which may take place over a number of meetings, the therapist will sit down with the person to agree on treatment goals. These might be aiming to see certain beliefs in a more rational way, or agreeing ways of dealing with abnormal perceptions such as hearing voices – for example, distraction techniques. Other treatment goals may include an increase in certain behaviours.

Regular sessions over many months are often needed, which will involve the therapist liaising closely with other members of the team to ensure that treatment approaches are carefully discussed and coordinated.

People with schizophrenia often experience depression and anxiety. The therapist may, therefore, help them with anxiety management training or a cognitive behavioural approach to improving mood, self-esteem and confidence.

Therapists will also identify particular areas of strength in the individual as it is important to emphasize that building strengths can sometimes be effective in reducing problems. For example, regardless of any illness we have, we all have areas of ability or areas where we have particular interests. Sarah's story illustrates this.

Sarah began to develop symptoms of schizophrenia while at university. She began her second year well, but by the end of the first term she had begun to develop worries that fellow students were recording her thoughts and broadcasting them to members of the 'secret service'. Because of these thoughts, Sarah became withdrawn and suspicious and stopped attending lectures. She also developed a fear that her food might be poisoned and thus became highly selective about what she would and would not eat. As a consequence she lost weight.

Eventually, Sarah went to see one of the university counsellors, who referred her to the student health service. The doctor in the student health service realized that Sarah was developing a significant mental health problem and referred her to a psychiatrist. A diagnosis of schizophrenia was made and Sarah started taking medication. It became clear that Sarah would be unable to resume her studies for the time being, and she returned to live with her family.

Over the next 2–3 months Sarah began to show some response to her medication and to the care provided by the local community mental health team. Sarah saw a community psychiatric nurse twice a week; this nurse encouraged Sarah to keep to a reasonable routine, to get up on time in the morning and generally to resume activities outside the house. Sarah became less suspicious and, through discussions with her community psychiatric nurse and psychiatrist, realized that she had an illness that would be helped by medication and that the thoughts she had about others were not real but part of the illness. Sarah's psychiatrist referred her to a clinical psychologist for CBT. Following an assessment it became clear that Sarah was still troubled by thoughts that others might do her some harm and that these thoughts were probably the greatest obstacle to Sarah returning to her previous social life. The psychologist was able to help Sarah challenge the thoughts she had about others wishing to cause her harm. The process included Sarah keeping a diary of her thoughts and in her sessions she was able to learn to counter her irrational thoughts with more rational beliefs.

From Sarah's file, her psychologist had noted that she was a good piano player. However, since starting university she had stopped playing, and although her parents had encouraged her to resume she had not shown any interest and her parents had just left it at that. Her psychologist realized that the illness had left Sarah in a state of very poor general confidence and that a process of confidence building would be an important element of her treatment, especially with respect to her long-term recovery. The psychologist therefore set out to reactivate Sarah's interest in piano playing, first of all by asking Sarah to play for him during one of her visits. Although Sarah realized she was 'rusty' it was clear that she still had her piano playing skills and she was pleased to see that the psychologist appreciated her skill. Over the next few weeks, with continued encouragement from the psychologist, Sarah was able to spend increasing periods of time practising the piano and was able to call one or two of her musical friends, who came over to the house with their musical instruments (a clarinet and a saxophone) to enjoy a happy musical evening.

Over the next few months Sarah eventually made a good recovery from her illness. Although she and her family were at times frustrated by what seemed to be slow progress, Sarah eventually resumed university studies and practised her piano playing for 1½ hours every day and, with her friends, had been able to play in public on a couple of occasions. Thus piano playing, with its consequent positive effects on her confidence, became an essential part of Sarah's treatment. The psychologist had correctly recognized that focusing solely on a person's problems is never enough; building on strengths can at least diminish the intensity of problems. It is also important to emphasize that from a professional point of view, simply focusing on problems hides a person's true identity and character.

## Creative therapies

It is a widely held belief that severe mental illness and enhanced creativity are related. However, the consensus of opinion among researchers who have studied this area suggest there is no link. Creative people are not more likely to be diagnosed with schizophrenia and people with schizophrenia are not more likely to be creative than mentally healthy people. Arts and creative therapies do, however, have therapeutic and social benefits and are recommended in the national treatment guidelines as an important addition to more traditional care such as medication and talking treatments. Arts therapies include art, dance, drama, creative writing and music. Practitioners are trained to postgraduate level and are registered with a professional body. Many mental health trusts employ art and music therapists or have access to independent community 'arts for health' projects.

Occasionally, the level of distress experienced by people with schizophrenia may hinder them in expressing themselves verbally. For them, writing creatively, using art materials and making or listening to music may be more therapeutic vehicles for self-expression and containing overwhelming feelings. Participating in creative therapies can improve confidence and self-esteem, and there is a growing evidence base for their role in improving negative symptoms. Despite people with mental health problems valuing such services and their positive impact on recovery and quality of life, these resources suffer from underfunding. Access to creative therapies will be dependent on where you live and information can usually be found in local mental health services directories. Some community art projects accept self-referrals, whereas a referral from your care coordinator or GP may be required for some services.

## Coping strategy for voices

At one time, professionals were taught to ignore the voices heard by people with schizophrenia because it was thought that, as much as possible, one should attempt to minimize their importance. However, as we learn more about the nature of these voices and their impact on the person who hears them, it has become clear that obtaining a clear picture of what the person is experiencing enables professionals and family members to help the person cope.

The first step is to ask the person to keep a diary of the voices, noting when and where they occur, and a detailed description of what the voices actually say. It is also important to help the person understand that voices are part of the illness and that they are actually misperceiving inner thoughts as coming from outside. When these thoughts are particularly distressing they sometimes indicate a wider degree of distress related to other thinking processes.

Voices may reduce or completely disappear if competing stimuli can be provided, such as relaxing music or the distraction of films or TV. Sometimes the person with schizophrenia becomes very frightened by the voices and it is therefore important to provide reassurance that the voices are simply a sign of the illness. The use of cognitive behavioural techniques to challenge the reality of voices is often helpful, and simple thought challenges may be taught to family members.

## Dealing with anger

Anger is an emotion that affects all of us to a greater or lesser degree. Some people, no matter what is said or done to them, do not become angry. Others – and we include people both with and without mental health problems – react to even the slightest provocation by becoming angry. Just witness an episode of road rage or go into a busy department store before Christmas! Most of us will have experienced anger when watching TV programmes depicting tragedies in developing countries or injustice of any kind. We become angry that the world is such a hard, cruel place for literally billions of people. Thus people with schizophrenia are, along with the rest of the population, entitled to become angry at times.

People with schizophrenia can also become angry because of their delusions and can simply become angry because of the problems caused by their illness. The most important thing is to let somebody know when you are feeling angry, so that you can discuss it and, if at all possible, resolve the situation. Some of the most effective methods of dealing with anger, other than discussion, are those that help reduce physical arousal, which underpins angry responses. Anxiety is a fight or flight reaction and so is anger, arising from an outpouring of adrenaline. Thus, simple methods such as physical relaxation and exercise are often useful in defusing angry episodes.

Any long-standing pattern of anger is something that you should be mention to your care coordinator or doctor so that you can receive help to deal with it – anger is one of the most unhelpful and unpleasant emotions that human beings experience.

## Dealing with depression

Depression is sometimes called, perhaps rather dismissively, the 'common cold' of psychiatry. Up to 20 per cent of the population will have a depressive episode at some time during their life. One pointer to its prevalence is the somewhat alarming statistic that in 2012 there were more than 40 million prescriptions for antidepressant drugs in the UK.

People with schizophrenia are even more likely to have depression than the general population. The causes of depression vary between individuals. It is likely that much depression in people with schizophrenia is due to biochemical factors, while the adverse consequences of the illness itself will inevitably lead to a depressed mood in many. So what can you do apart from take antidepressant medication? There are several proven non-drug treatments for depression, which are well described in the NICE guidelines. These are:

- Behavioural activation
- Computerized cognitive behavioural therapy
- Physical activity (see Chapter 15).

### Behavioural activation

Behavioural activation is defined as 'a treatment in which the person with depression and the therapist work together to identify the effect of behaviour on symptoms, feelings and problems'. It encourages people to develop more positive behaviour such as planning activities and doing constructive things that they would usually avoid. Lack of activity is a common problem for people with schizophrenia and is probably one of the most common causes of depression for people with the illness.

An excellent self-help book written for those with depression is *Manage Your Mood: How to Use Behavioural Activation Techniques to Overcome Depression* by David Veale and Robert Willson. There are also a number of helpful descriptions of behavioural activation on YouTube. One helpful, brief video features Dr Kevin Arnold, psychologist from the world-famous Center for Cognitive and Behavioural Therapy of Greater Columbus <http://www.youtube.com/watch?v=Dp6i3GUasqQ>. As you probably know, YouTube has become an excellent source of information although, as with most things on the Internet, you need to be somewhat cautious about what you watch!

It is encouraging to note that many more mental health professionals are now trained to use behavioural activation, and if you have depression and this has not been offered to you, you should ask – perhaps suggesting that your care coordinator has a look at this book!

## Computerized cognitive behavioural therapy (CCBT)

CCBT, originally developed some 25 years ago, is now widely used in the NHS. Research shows that it can be helpful for a range of conditions, notably anxiety, phobias, obsessive–compulsive disorder and depression. Research also shows that it is most effective when there is some guidance from a professional. All of us need support and encouragement, and if you are keen to try CCBT you should let your care coordinator know so that you can be provided with suitable support and advice.

One of the best programmes available is MoodGYM <www. moodgym.anu.edu.au>. It is completely without charge; just log in and give it a try. As the name suggests, this programme is primarily for those with depression. However, anyone with problems relating to self-esteem or poor self-image will benefit.

## Relaxation

Although relaxation is not used directly as a treatment for schizophrenia, it can be helpful in reducing the general level of physical tension, anxiety and general arousal, which often lead to distress. The instructions that follow will give you an introduction if you want to have a try. Otherwise, there are various relaxation exercises available on CD or in other forms.

While there are many ways to achieve relaxation, most focus on a systematic tensing and relaxing of the muscles in the body. This has two benefits. First, it helps you to differentiate between states of tension and relaxation and, importantly, recognize when your level of muscle tension is increasing. Second, there is considerable evidence to suggest that systematic tensing and relaxing exercises eventually lead to a state of overall muscle relaxation and, as a consequence, a feeling of well-being.

The following instructions are straightforward. It may be helpful to read and inwardly digest them, then make a recording that you can follow. If you do this, however, remember to leave a 10-second gap between each phase. This may be as effective as any commercially available recording and is certainly worth trying, as unlike them it is free!

First of all, identify a time in the day when you have 30 minutes to devote to the task. Find a quiet room, unplug the phone and turn off your mobile, and wear loose, comfortable clothing. The exercise can be carried out in a comfortable chair or lying down, and you should experiment with different situations and times of the day to identify what the optimum conditions are for you.

Before doing the exercises it is important to remember to tense your muscles only to a moderate extent. If you tense them too hard you will defeat the object of the exercise. A simple guide is that it should lead to no more than a sensation of tensing or 'pulling'; if you experience pain you are trying too hard. Furthermore, when you release the tension you should feel it go immediately.

> Get in position and begin with your right hand. Clench your fist so that your knuckles are white. Hold for 5 seconds, then release immediately.
> *Pause, wait 10 seconds, then repeat.*
>
> Tense your right forearm, closing your fist and tensing the muscles of your forearm. Remember, not too hard. Hold for 5 seconds, then release immediately.
> *Pause, wait 10 seconds, then repeat.*
>
> Tense your right biceps, clenching your fist and bending your arm so that it forms a 90° angle. Concentrate on making your biceps bulge as much as possible. Hold for 5 seconds, then release immediately.
> *Pause, wait 10 seconds, then repeat.*
>
> Repeat these actions with the left hand, forearm and biceps. Remembering to do each exercise twice, hold for 5 seconds, then release immediately.
>
> Next move your head and neck. Tense your eye muscles. Screw up your eyes and keep them shut tight. Hold for 5 seconds, then release immediately.
> *Pause, wait 10 seconds, then repeat.*
>
> Tense your mouth by clenching your jaws together and concentrate on pressing your lips together as firmly as possible. At the same time you will notice that you tense your eyes. Hold for 5 seconds, then release immediately.
> *Pause, wait 10 seconds, then repeat.*
>
> Now concentrate on tensing your neck. Push your chin down a little towards your chest but do not touch your chest. Hold for 5 seconds, then release immediately.
> *Pause, wait 10 seconds, then repeat.*

Next, move your shoulders and back, pushing your shoulders up slightly and tensing your neck. Feel the muscles tighten across your shoulders. Hold for 5 seconds, then release immediately.
*Pause, wait 10 seconds, then repeat.*

Tense your shoulders and arms by pushing your arms down, holding your neck rigid. Concentrate on tensing across your shoulders. Hold for 5 seconds, then release immediately.
*Pause, wait 10 seconds, then repeat.*

Tense the muscles in your back by pushing your elbows into your sides, pulling your shoulders down, holding your neck tight and pushing your head down towards your chest. Concentrate on tensing the muscles across your back. Hold for 5 seconds, then release immediately.
*Pause, wait 10 seconds, then repeat.*

Now move to your chest and abdomen. Tense the muscles of your chest by pushing your shoulders back, pushing your elbows down into your waist and tilting your head back slightly and concentrate on holding your chest in a barrel-like, rigid way. Hold for 5 seconds, then release immediately.
*Pause, wait 10 seconds, then repeat.*

Tense the muscles of your stomach from the back and pull in towards your navel. Hold for 5 seconds, then release immediately.
*Pause, wait 10 seconds, then repeat.*

Next, move to your lower body and legs. Tense your thighs and buttocks by pushing your buttocks down and concentrate on tensing your thighs and buttocks together. Hold for 5 seconds, then release immediately.
*Pause, wait 10 seconds, then repeat.*

Tense your right calf by pulling your toes up towards you, keeping your leg straight at the knee. Pull your toes back until you can feel the pull all the way up your calf muscles. Hold for 5 seconds, then release immediately.
*Pause, wait 10 seconds, then repeat.*

Tense your right foot by curling over your toes, trying to make your toes clench like a fist. Hold for 5 seconds, then release immediately.
*Pause, wait 10 seconds, then repeat.*

Repeat this sequence for your left calf and foot.

When you come to this point, begin to tense your whole body, starting with your hands, working up through your arms, then your head, neck, shoulders, back, chest, stomach, buttocks, thighs, calves and feet. Take 10 seconds to gradually tense the whole body. Hold for 5 seconds, then relax.

As you relax, slowly breathe out as much as you can. Keep your eyes closed and say 'calm' to yourself.

Repeat this sequence five times, remembering to leave 10 seconds between each.

Next, concentrate on slowing down your breathing. Try to use all of your chest and, as you breathe out, say 'calm' to yourself. Let your breathing settle into a natural rhythm and then try to fix your mind on a quiet and relaxing scene. Imagine yourself lying on a beach or in a meadow. Imagine a warm atmosphere around you. Try to image the smells of this environment. Keep your mind as fixed on this place as possible and let yourself drift. Don't worry if you fall asleep, but perhaps it may be worth setting your alarm clock first!

## Breathing exercises

Breathing exercises are probably one of the most effective ways of dealing with high levels of anxiety, and they are also helpful at times when you simply need to calm down. Controlling your breathing not only gives you a feeling of calm but also reduces your blood pressure and generally reduces stress on the body. Remember that breathing should involve all the chest and diaphragm. Breathing from the top of the chest – the anxious breathing that we all experience at times – promotes more anxiety.

### Simple exercises

One of the most important things about controlled breathing is to slow down your breathing rate gradually, so that eventually you are breathing 6–8 times a minute, instead of 14, 16 or more. Simply find somewhere to relax – and a nice comfortable chair is better than a bed – put one hand at the top of your chest and the other hand on your upper abdomen. Breathe in through your nose, making sure that the whole chest inflates. You can feel this by the movement in your hands. Breathe very slowly in. Hold it and then exhale slowly.

Another trick that is often used is alternate nostril breathing, something that is often practised in yoga classes. Sit for a while in a comfortable chair and relax as much as possible. Then, place your right thumb over your right nostril and breathe in through your left nostril. When you have taken in a deep breath, close off your left nostril and exhale through your right nostril. Continue this breathing for 5–10 minutes – it really works. Breathing exercises often work well after you have practised deep muscle relaxation techniques. Many people advocate using a breathing or relaxation technique twice a day. Although this may take up 45 minutes or so, you will find that for the rest of the day you feel much calmer, and actually your efficiency in everyday tasks will be increased if you are more relaxed.

## Family therapy

When schizophrenia presents as a long-term illness, the affected person tends to spend a great amount of time in close proximity to the family, as with any chronic illness. We know from the wide range of research, carried out not only on schizophrenia, that this close proximity may often cause a negative atmosphere, which can often be exacerbated by family members taking a critical attitude to the manifestations of illness, such as apathy and withdrawal. Unless family members recognize that apathy and withdrawal are actually signs of illness, rather than just signs of laziness, it is easy to understand how critical comments and a negative family atmosphere may arise. Eventually, this may lead to an increase in stress for the affected person and thus increase the severity of their illness.

It is therefore important that a comprehensive assessment of the family is undertaken by the care coordinator or other member of the multidisciplinary team. The assessment will look at the family structure and various relationships within the family. It is also important that it considers the cultural context of the family. Mental health professionals need to understand that family structures are different in different cultures, and what would be acceptable in one culture may be unacceptable in another. Therefore, the assessment needs to be undertaken with considerable sensitivity.

Another important issue in assessment is to establish exactly what family members know about the schizophrenic illness.

## Mental health consequences of schizophrenia for family members

There is now a great deal of research that suggests that caring for someone with a long-term illness, either physical or mental, leads to an increased chance of depression, anxiety or other mental health problems in carers. Mental health professionals and the GP need to be aware that family members are especially vulnerable. Once more, it is an important part of the Care Programme Approach to identify the needs of carers as well as those of the affected person. It is thus important to identify the mental health needs of family members and to ensure that they receive any necessary care and treatment.

### Family interventions

Unfortunately, in times gone by, families were often blamed for causing schizophrenia. These now discredited theories are remembered by older mental health professionals with great shame. From blaming families, we have now come to acknowledge that they often bear a tremendous burden when one of their members develops a schizophrenic illness. In the past three decades we have identified some specific interventions that now meet many of the needs of family members.

In our opinion, the first priority is to ensure that family members are provided with practical help and support and that they access the correct benefits from an increasingly complex system. Family members can provide an enormous amount of unpaid care and often do not claim the benefits to which they are entitled. It is also important that family members are provided with as much practical support as possible, and the care coordinator should identify these needs.

Apart from practical ways of helping the family, there is now a range of helpful interventions, which if targeted to the family as a whole – including the person with schizophrenia – provide benefits to all.

Interventions can only begin when the professional involved gets to know the family well and has established a rapport. Describing family interventions in detail is not possible within the confines of this book, but there are some excellent texts, primarily written for mental health professionals, comprehensible to the average lay reader. For further detail we recommend an excellent book written by two psychologists and a psychiatrist who have not only researched this area but also worked with many families: *Family Work for Schizophrenia: A Practical Guide* by Elizabeth Kuipers *et al.*

Family interventions often need to take place over many months and are quite consuming of mental health professionals' time. However, there is plenty of research that shows that time spent with the family is a good investment, as when family interventions are carried out well over a reasonable period of time, they assist with keeping the affected person well and appear to reduce the frequency of relapse.

# Part 3
# FURTHER HELP

# 9

# Sources of practical help

## Advocates and advocacy services

Many people with schizophrenia need others to speak for them on occasion, as their illness may result in them being unable adequately to express their wishes and needs. Someone might thus be needed to speak on the individual's behalf when communicating with the clinical team about treatment issues such as medication or psychological therapy. For those receiving inpatient care, advocates can perform a wide range of valuable roles – everything from ensuring that the individual is receiving an appropriate diet to making sure that, where necessary, they have access to the correct advice regarding benefits and housing matters.

Services in the UK are committed to ensuring that those in need of an advocate, notably people without the support of carers and family members, are provided with an appropriate service. Many advocates have had a mental health problem themselves and thus have valuable insights into what mental health services have to offer and the problems and pitfalls of being a 'patient'.

Mental health services have budgets from which to employ advocates, either directly or through self-help organizations. Advocates are independent of the clinical team and operate within the usual codes of conduct expected with regard to privacy and confidentiality.

There are a number of organizations that provide advocacy services, such as Rethink Mental Illness. To quote from its website <www.rethink.org>:

> Our advocacy services are designed to support those who are vulnerable or need help to make informed decisions and secure the rights and services to which they are entitled. We have a great deal of experience in developing and delivering quality advocacy services across a variety of settings, both in the community and in secure hospitals and secure units.

Mind <www.mind.org.uk> also provides a wide range of independent advice and information.

## Citizens Advice Bureaux

Citizens Advice Bureaux (CAB) are perhaps the most important
sources of free help and advice for people with schizophrenia,
on a wide range of matters, from help navigating an increasingly
complex benefits system, to housing, employment and advice for
those in debt. CAB advisers have received specialist training in a
range of matters and operate with the highest standards of confidentiality. Some CAB offices have the services of legally qualified
advisers, most of whom work on a voluntary (unpaid) basis. In
addition to giving free advice, CAB can help with filling out forms
and, where necessary, dealing with creditors directly. They may also
draft papers for you in courts and tribunals and may, on occasion,
help you to present your case.

In these days of austerity, where access to legal advice is becoming
more restricted, CAB perform an invaluable function in assisting
those in society without the means to employ lawyers or seek
advice for which payment is required.

## Money advice services

It has been estimated that 1 in 4 people with a mental health
problem also has a debt problem.

In a survey by the Money Advice Trust and the Royal College of
Psychiatrists in November 2010, 1,270 frontline staff in creditor and
debt collection agencies were surveyed. It was found that roughly
half of all debtors also had a mental health problem. Mental health
problems can be both the result and cause of problems with debt.

Debt is the second most popular area of enquiry, after benefits,
for CAB, which deal with a large number of cases nationally each
year. There are a further three national charities that provide free
debt advice. These are National Debtline, StepChange Debt Charity
and Payplan. All can assist you in choosing the right strategy for
dealing with debts, such as a debt management plan, debt relief
order, individual voluntary arrangement or bankruptcy, enabling
you to choose an option that is suitable for your situation and

income, and to make realistic offers of payment. A money adviser will go through your debts and help draw up a financial statement of income and expenditure. The financial statement identifies areas where it may be possible to make savings, freeing up money to spend on necessities such as food, rent and participation in social activities. The priority is protecting your home, fuel supply and liberty before dealing with the less urgent debts such as credit card and catalogue debts. A money adviser will also explore ways of boosting income, such as claiming Personal Independence Payments (PIPs), which are gradually replacing Disability Living Allowance between 2013 and 2016.

The Debt and Mental Health Evidence Form was created in 2007 as part of a joint initiative between the Money Advice Trust and the Royal College of Psychiatrists. The form enables an organization giving money advice (such as CAB) to use evidence from a health care professional to notify creditors of the client's mental health problem, with the client's consent. This ensures that a creditor or a collector engages the advice agency and the client in a way that takes account of any mental health problems. For example, it may be important not to contact the client by telephone, if they have difficulty using one. This process may also be used to negotiate options such a final settlement at a reduced rate and, in a small number of cases, a complete write-off of the debt.

# 10

## The law

### The Mental Health Act (1983)

In our opinion, it is essential that people with schizophrenia and their families know about the Mental Health Act and its various components. Unfortunately, a minority of people with schizophrenia become so ill that they require admission to hospital under a 'section'. We need to emphasize that applying a section is a last resort and only used where there is real risk to the person or others and when he or she refuses voluntary admission. We cannot provide a comprehensive account of what is quite complex legislation but it is important to explain some of the important facts about the Act.

Once again, we want to emphasize that the legislation is underpinned by the principle of providing care in the least restrictive manner and the admission of a person to hospital against his or her will should therefore be seen as a last resort. An application for the admission of a person to hospital under a section requires an assessment by a specialist social worker, the GP and psychiatrist and, where possible, family members are involved. Usually, initial admission to hospital is for a short period of 72 hours, so that assessment may take place. It is only after this, if it is appropriate and in the person's best interests, that an application is made to detain them for longer, either for a period of further assessment of 28 days or, eventually, a period of treatment of 6 months.

It is important to emphasize that the person has the right to appeal against their detention. Such appeals are held by a Mental Health Act Tribunal, which normally consists of a judge, a psychiatrist not connected with the particular service where the person is being detained, and another lay member who is independent of the hospital and others involved in the case.

It is also worth emphasizing that tribunals commonly uphold appeals. The Act is set out in such a way that detained people are provided with a full description of their rights once the section has been completed and mental health services are obliged to assist as far as possible with the process of appealing. In this case, mental health services have to ensure that the person has an advocate if needed; this being a family member or friend or an independent advocate from one of the advocacy services, who may or may not be connected with the hospital where the person is being detained.

People detained under the Act have a range of rights and safeguards, and in addition to the right to appeal, the various treatments offered to them are subject to approval by a 'second opinion appointed doctor' – a doctor who is independent of that particular service, who carries out in his or her own right an assessment of the patient and either agrees or disagrees with the treatment being proposed by the patient's consultant.

## Mental Health Review Tribunals

Mental Health Review Tribunals are independent bodies that are set up under the Mental Health Act and, in the same way as Employment Tribunals, have legal powers. Tribunals consist of three individuals: a judge who acts as the chair, a lay member and a medical member. All those detained under the Mental Health Act have the right to apply to a Mental Health Review Tribunal to have their detention reviewed. The appeal process is the same as for other legal processes. Anyone appealing against a detention is therefore entitled to legal representation. This is paid for by the Legal Services Commission. Each hospital will provide assistance with a list of solicitors who are approved to act in tribunal cases and the Mental Health Review Tribunal Office will also supply a list of approved solicitors. The Tribunal Office will ensure that the hearing is convenient to the detained person and that he or she is independently examined by the tribunal doctor. The person is entitled to call witnesses on his or her behalf and solicitors will be helpful in identifying what evidence is needed. The tribunal may overturn the detention and has the power to order the discharge of the patient into the community.

## Other legislation and rights

It is important to emphasize that people with schizophrenia and their families are just as entitled to protection under law as any other member of society. Therefore, there is an entitlement to legal representation if you cannot afford to pay for your own, there is the right to speak to your MP and, with regard to treatment from health services, there is the right to ask the Health Ombudsman to intervene on your behalf: <www.ombudsman.org.uk>. All modern mental health services have a policy of ensuring that those with schizophrenia and their families are given plentiful information regarding their rights, and that practical support and help will be readily available to all those who require it.

Of particular importance to people with schizophrenia is the Disability Discrimination Act, which was passed in 1995. This Act has now been subsumed into the Equality Act of 2010, and you can find information about disability, whether physical or mental, on the government's website <www.gov.uk/browse/disabilities>. Anyone with a long-term illness such as schizophrenia will be covered by the Equality Act. This provides them with protection in respect of housing, employment and – more generally – gives them access to equal opportunities within society.

Some people with long-term conditions can also be protected in some circumstances by the Court of Protection. Individuals whose illness is so severe that they lack the capacity to decide important matters for themselves regarding finances, making a will etc. may be protected by a family member who assumes power of attorney or, in some cases, the Court of Protection. This is based in the Royal Courts of Justice and is an institution set up by government to make decisions and appoint deputies on behalf of people who are unable to make decisions about their personal health, finance or welfare. We emphasize that most people with schizophrenia, even those who may have an active form of their illness, are able to make choices about where they live and how they spend their money. Unless the illness is very severe, all professionals know that people with schizophrenia have the right to live their lives as anyone else in society.

Turning back to the myths referred to at the start of Chapter 5, UK law is such that the rights of individuals with mental illnesses are well protected and only in exceptional circumstances are their rights to live a normal life taken away – and then for the shortest period of time possible.

# 11

## Austin's story and a carer's perspective

We thought long and hard about the presentation of this book. We decided that we should use real stories from those who know best: 'Austin's story' is the account of someone with schizophrenia and 'Georgie's story' is a commentary by someone who cares for a person with schizophrenia. It is our view that publishing these stories is the best way of conveying the reality of this devastating illness.

### Austin's story

My name is Austin Thompson, I'm 22 and am currently holding down two jobs. I first began hearing voices when I was 12 or 13; I can't pinpoint an exact date or event that first triggered them. All I know is that around that time I was acting aggressively and errati- cally in response to a number of things, including my parents' very public divorce. The voices, two of them, would keep me awake at night and I'd often react to them during the day; one voice would say my name, or part of my name, especially when I was in crowded areas. This only increased my growing sense that I was being fol- lowed and watched. The second voice would criticize me and what I was doing; this was very depressing, to say the least.

Not knowing how to react to these voices, I decided not to seek help and to deal with them privately. Perhaps I was afraid of what would happen should anyone know about them. Only when I was 15 did I accept help and even then I felt the person I spoke to didn't believe me. However, this could have been my paranoia about accepting help in the first place. This help came after a violent outburst that came out of nowhere, causing a deeply regretful altercation – I'm thankful that no one was hurt. I then went to counselling, but I wasn't ready for it yet and therefore didn't see the value in it. After all, I had dealt with the voices for this long with only one outburst. The counselling sessions didn't last long and when they finished there was no follow up or referral. Therefore I went back to being on my own with these two voices in my head.

I can't remember when I learned to stop worrying and accept the voices as part of who I was. However, I assume that it must have been around the time I went to college. I saw these voices as part of me. They were something no one else could hear and that annoyed me from time to time. However, they still belonged to me. Around this time I came up with the name 'Constant Companion' to describe whatever was wrong with me – the voices and the paranoia; all these things were now one entity that had a name. I don't know what I wanted to achieve by humanizing it, but it helped when I became frustrated with it.

I don't wish to sour anyone against romantic relationships so I won't speak too in-depth about mine. However, I should mention that I was in a relationship for 3 years and it ended badly for me. When I went to university and my routine was thrown out of the window, my Constant Companion went wild. My girl-friend at the time tried her best to tell me how important it was for my own health that I continue with my routine. However, I wasn't ready to listen to someone tell me what to do with this new-found freedom, even though she loved me. In the end she couldn't handle my increasingly erratic behaviour and decided to end things. The months that followed are a blur of not sleeping, drinking, taking any kind of drug I could find, and hurting people who just wanted to help me. I choose not to look back on this time, as I know that I handled it badly and my Constant Companion took hold. I made an attempt on my own life by overdosing on diazepam. Thankfully I survived, possibly down to the large amount of stimulants I had taken. However, I can't stress how lucky I am to be alive.

After the attempted overdose I was put in contact with Bournemouth's Early Intervention Team, though after 7 years of dealing with my Constant Companion did I really qualify for 'early' intervention? They did their best, but in the end I dropped out of university. The environment was wrong for me to continue, what with the pressures of living by myself for the first time with only one or two real friends who I could rely on.

I moved back home to live with my brother, sister and mother. Having my mother's support has meant the world to me. Even if she doesn't fully understand my illness she has always been there for me. My siblings never ask questions about my Constant Companion, and while it means I'm never sure how they feel about it, it also means that I think they've accepted it. This acceptance, though quiet and understated, is what I look for in all my relationships, be they romantic, familial or platonic. The best advice I could give people whose loved ones have any mental health issues would be that they be calm, understanding and patient.

Since the move home I have started taking medication, something I fought against for a long time. For a while I viewed it as giving up on myself and letting something else control what was wrong with me. No longer do I feel this way. Medication is merely a tool in the kit of recovery. It isn't some miracle cure, a pill that you can take whenever you feel bad and 'boom' you're cured for a while. It's a part of stabilizing you, so that you can focus on the rest of the things needed to become happy and confident enough to do it yourself. For a while, in my dark days of university, I chose to medicate myself with alcohol and stimulants, none of which helped in any way other than to temporarily alleviate the Companion before it came back with greater force. It was an easy mistake and a quick fix, a temporary high for a long-term low, and though it has been tempting to go back to those ways, I won't because of the damage I did to myself and to those around me.

As I mentioned before, I have humanized my illness – I call it my Constant Companion. This encapsulates both the regular two voices that I hear and my paranoia. During times of extreme stress, or after long periods without sleep and without medication, my Companion changes and becomes something that requires a great deal of effort to control again – movements in shadows or out of the corner of my eye, hearing other voices of people I know, talking and arguing with myself at length, getting lost in thoughts that jump from one seemingly random topic to another, and hearing music. When these 'blips' (as one of the Richmond Early Intervention Team called them) occur, it takes me weeks to get over them. I can do this by seriously focusing on my routine and actively clinging onto normality. When the blips happen I find it comforting to tell myself, 'You have done something to your brain, relax, it will pass', and it does after a time, until I'm just left with the two voices.

Everyone has their own triggers, things that can set off unmanageable hallucinations. With the Richmond Early Intervention Team I worked out mine – things like prolonged use of stimulants (both legal and illegal), lack of sleep and ambiguous situations – to name a few. By recognizing what my triggers are I have learned not only to avoid them but also how to deal with them, as is the case with ambiguous situations, which can't always be avoided.

The methods I have found helpful for coping with the two voices and the feelings of paranoia and emotional numbness that go with them are:

*Controlled breathing*  I don't mean meditation. That may work for some people but not for me. I mean taking a minute to acknowledge the voices and mentally tell them to be quiet. It's hard to do, even though it sounds easy, especially as you have to keep it internal, lest you freak out a quiet bus by yelling 'Shut up!' I have found that smoking calms me, though I believe it to be the breathing pattern of smoking and not the actual tobacco itself. Nicotine is a stimulant, after all, and I am always aware that the frequency with which I smoke makes things worse rather than better.

*Regular sleep*  For me, sleep is a big trigger. I know this and I try to keep it as a top priority. Remember, nothing good happens after 2.00 a.m. so why stick around to see it? I should also stress that sleeping the day away isn't going to be helpful for coping or indeed thriving with your own Constant Companion; you need to keep active.

*Routine*  Simple things like regular washing, brushing teeth and going food shopping often got forgotten when I was at some of my worst times. An inexplicable fear of showering was one of my problems and made my presence unpleasant for others. While being able to be alone is a big step in coping, being able to be around friends and co-workers should be the ultimate goal. A routine helps focus your mind, especially in the mornings and evenings (when the mind is either fresh or preparing for sleep).

*Support*  Though I had to deal with my voices and all that goes with them alone for a long time, I didn't have to. I found that once

I accepted the voices as part of myself, I could open up to people I trusted and I found their love and support a major boon to keeping calm and controlling my Constant Companion. Support can be from anyone who has your best interests at heart: friends, loved ones, family and even doctors. It can be hard to trust doctors or medical professionals, like it is hard to trust anyone sometimes. However, be assured that I have found people to generally exceed my expectations when it comes to understanding my illness and the way I deal with it. Sharing my feelings about my Constant Companion has been hard for me to do, but the more support I've found in the people around me, the easier it has been for me to open up, which I think is a big step in coping.

*Set yourself goals*  Every year on my birthday I make a list of the things I would like to accomplish in the year. I started doing this the year I dropped out of university; nothing huge and unobtainable, but small things like not having another blip, avoiding drugs and learning to drive. These were small, manageable goals on a road to being happy with myself. Above all else it helped me put my Constant Companion to one side and focus on other areas of my life, because if I let my illness take control of my life I would never be able to grow and get past it. I'd be another person who let something that is negative and beyond their control define them. That's how I see it anyway.

It sounds strange, but I do feel lonely sometimes when I don't have my Constant Companion with me. For example, I didn't have my Constant Companion with me when I first started on medication. I was very drowsy and spent most of my time asleep or with family. I guess that is normal for someone who has learned to live with unaided hallucinations regularly. Looking back, I should have savoured those moments of silence and calm and used them as a mental base to think back on when things began to be hectic.

I have had good friends, ones that understood my illness, and others who didn't know how to react to it and so chose to do some things that didn't help at all. One example was at university, when I was home for the weekend and left my room door unlocked. My housemates and 'friends' decided it would be a good idea to take my sheets off my bed and set them on fire in the courtyard. You can imagine what the voices were saying to me when I found out.

These were not good friends and I wish that I had seen the signs earlier and avoided being stuck with these people. However, not all my friendship groups have been so destructive. Returning home after leaving university, while still battling a very bad time with my Constant Companion, I made friends with some students local to me. This was helpful as they are the most understanding and caring people I could have hoped to meet; they've put up with me asking if they heard something I'm sure was in my head. They've allowed me to act like myself, without the fear of judgement. I do frequently check that I'm not bothering them with being around and apologize for any behaviour I think they might find strange or unsettling. However, I'm always told to not worry about it. I do wonder what my life would have been like had I met these people at university.

Despite the sometimes crippling paranoia I do thrive from being around other people. I have always surrounded myself with people, good or bad for me. My oldest friends, those I've had in my life since I was 9 years old, can remember me from a time before my illness and, though it's hard for everyone to grow and change, they have been there for me even when I've pushed them away. They know that I am still essentially the same person I have always been. It has been a lot of work keeping these friends. Life has a tendency to drag those close to you away, and I have lost touch with people whom I was close to and it has been hard. I do question whether perhaps the way I've acted because of my Constant Companion has driven certain people away. However, you can't do that; you can't go down that road – it leads to dark thoughts about yourself and this has to be avoided. I often hear the lower voice saying things like, 'They're talking about you' or 'They hate you', especially around groups of people I don't know or trust. The voices you hear are part of you; they are your thoughts, even if they seem so external. They are so haphazard that at times it's easier to pass them off as something beyond you. I remember speaking to a member of the early intervention team about the difference between fact and opinion. What I took away from it was that the voices in my head aren't perfect; they are part of me and as such are like me in that they have opinions. All opinions can be argued against. I found that actually arguing with the lower voice seemed to agitate it and make it louder. However, simply knowing that the voices aren't always right means that I can choose to ignore them more easily than if I view them as always correct.

It's hard to think of my life 10 years ago, before my Constant Companion, and I think I miss it. However, my life now is something I'm happy with. Though I may not have travelled the path I thought I would, I'm still grateful for the one I'm on and for the people who are there to guide, love and support me along it.

## Georgie's story

### The early years

Our youngest son, Christian, developed paranoid schizophrenia at the age of 16; he is now 39. To say that this was a shock is an understatement; we were traumatized, grieving and totally disbelieving. My name is Georgie; my husband Paul and I have been carers for 23 years. For the first 7 years Christian lived with us in our home, and life for all of us was painful and extremely difficult.

Christian had always been an outgoing boy. The illness came on subtly and slowly and it was hard to detect how much was raging hormones and normal teenage behaviour and how much was something far more sinister. He started having problems concentrating at school. He became argumentative and stroppy at home, like many teenagers. However, what I believe escalated his behaviour was when Christian and his friend were returning home after a day's shopping, when they were held at knifepoint on a train by a man who had been let out of prison a few days before. He told them they would be dead by the time they reached the next station. When Christian came home he visibly shook for the next 3 days. His friend's father, who is a pharmacist, knocked on my door and said, 'Watch your son; my son is fine but yours isn't, he's been traumatized.'

Following this event, Christian's life took a different direction. He became increasingly reclusive and refused to sit at the dinner table; he would insist on taking his food to his bedroom and eating in there. One day he stood in the middle of the lawn in torrential rain for over an hour. His hair was stuck to his face, his clothes soaked through: he didn't seem to know what to do, where to go or even who he was. Remarkably, he had a couple of jobs after leaving school but struggled with his concentration. He started throwing clothes away that had patterns on them because he thought they interfered with his concentration. He would be scared that his friends would break in and harm us.

Nowadays there are early intervention teams to ensure that things run far more smoothly, saving families from the anxiety that we were forced to go through. But early intervention was unheard of in those days. Getting help for Christian took 14 months and three appointments with his GP, who seemed to think that I was over-reacting. The first two times I went to see him he was unhelpful and dismissive.

Luckily a friend came with me the third time and, with her support and backup, our GP finally agreed to send two social workers to assess Christian. By now he weighed just over 8 stone and at 6 feet 2 inches tall was little more than skin and bone.

## The wilderness years

We spent the next 9 years in the wilderness. Christian was pre-scribed medication. No one explained to us what it was or what it was supposed to achieve. We thought he'd be his old self in a few weeks. No one really told us what was wrong with him. The psychiatrist told us he had a 'thought pattern disorder'. He would talk 'gobbledygook', or his words would be a jumble whereby nothing made any sense, but no one thought to explain 'thought disorder' to us. The confusion this caused (high expressed emotion, as the professionals refer to it) could easily have been avoided had someone thought to give us some kind of explanation. Our son had changed from being an extremely articulate, witty and highly intelligent young man into someone who was unable even to follow a conversation. We needed to understand thought disorder, auditory hallucinations, visual hal-lucinations, thought block, etc. – so-called 'positive' symptoms. We also needed to be told about the inertia, total lack of interest and the endless sleeping caused by the medication – we were not warned about the effects of that.

In place of the old Christian another son appeared, one who slept constantly and walked around like a zombie with lead boots on. I foolishly believed that he would just get up one day and the son we used to know would miraculously reappear. Owing to our total lack of understanding, I would for example run a bath and try to force him to get in it. I would try to get him friends and part-time work, but I could not see that he was incapable of doing these things.

It was my sister who first suggested, some 6 years after he became ill, that Chris had paranoid schizophrenia, after discussing his case and medication with a psychiatrist she knew. I refused to accept this and insisted she was wrong, believing that surely the doctors would have told me! It was only when we applied for benefits 6 or 7 years into his illness and a letter came through that said, 'Mr Christian John Wakefield has paranoid schizophrenia', that we had what might be called a proper diagnosis. I remember dropping the letter. I was in a daze. The GP later said to me, 'Well, you did realize he had schizophrenia, didn't you?' I honestly didn't. No one had ever told us. Hindsight is a great thing. Perhaps the GP and psychiatrist didn't tell us because of fears about the impact the diagnosis would have on us all. However, 'protecting' us in this way just delayed the inevitable. Being starved of valuable information meant the well-meaning things we were doing as a family were sometimes making the situation worse.

The next few years were spent either in hospital or in 24-hour care. Christian and the rest of the family had no quality of life. We just existed. Relationships with other family members deteriorated. The illness consumes you. It infects you. You think, 'Why my son?' I do think that the younger people develop this condition the poorer the prognosis might be, simply because the older you are at its onset, the more you have to fall back on in recovery. Christian had no experience of the working world, relationships, driving a car and so on, and consequently it's almost as if he hasn't evolved at the normal rate and is caught up in a kind of time warp. I would get frustrated with practitioners. I vividly remember Christian's nurse saying, 'Mrs Wakefield, try going to college, you could do music or art'. I was thinking, 'How on earth do you think I could go to college and concentrate when my teenage son is losing his mind before my very eyes?'

We faced many experiences of stigma. Vandals smashed all the security lights around the building of his new supported accommodation the night it opened. In another incident, a local head teacher called the police when she saw Christian sitting by the side of the swimming pool trying to decide whether to get in or not. It's hard to believe that in this day and age, someone in her position had so little knowledge of mental illness. The media do not help our situation. They use derogatory words such as 'schizo' and 'psycho', which fuels the embers of ignorance about our plight.

## Recovery or discovery?

After a painfully long wait I have finally accepted the fact that there is only so much that we as parents can do and that, for our son, there is no cure for schizophrenia. Having said that, we will never stop fighting his corner or indeed missing the son he was before this dreadful illness tore into all of our lives. Christian takes 500 mg of clozapine daily – this drug is the gold standard for treatment-resistant schizophrenia. It tends to work where all else fails and his condition did improve greatly after he was prescribed it. Within 12 weeks he moved from 24-hour to 12-hour care. Sadly, this was only prescribed 9 years into his illness. Had he received it earlier, as I understand happens at some hospitals, he might have been spared years of mental torture, and us years of anxiety and heartache. This thought haunts me – would he have recovered to a far better level had I known about this drug? A loaded question and one to which I will never know the answer. Again, this is a demonstration of the lack of information faced by carers and people with schizophrenia.

Christian's cognitive functioning is still poor. He can't think on his feet, which causes him many problems. For example, he will often go into a shop, fill his basket with groceries and then realize that he hasn't got any money, which makes him feel embarrassed and ashamed. He will put a pizza in the microwave for too long and when it explodes and sticks to the roof he will panic and not know what to do, other than call me to help him. Christian still suffers from both auditory and visual hallucinations, his thoughts are often disordered and he also gets thought broadcast, which convinces him that people can actually hear what he is thinking; or he often says that the people on TV know everything about him. This means that his confidence is at an all-time low.

Sometimes it can mean prompting him to do things, as he is so preoccupied with what goes on in his mind. Christian's mental health fluctuates regularly and dramatically throughout the day and this prevents him from doing everyday personal tasks; for example, sometimes he needs gently reminding about his washing and general hygiene routine, to get up and be motivated to face the day, to keep appointments for blood tests or to see his GP or consultant psychiatrist. However, this is not to the same degree as before he was prescribed clozapine. I see his recovery to date as a combination of so many factors. He has learned what to welcome and what to avoid. This goes for us as his carers too; we have all learned many lessons along the way. You can use the word recovery but the key to managing this condition is more about discovery, because discovering how to deal with schizophrenia is imperative to the whole family unit.

The next key stage in the family's recovery was when Christian employed a personal assistant through the government's personal budgets scheme, designed to provide funding for things that will improve quality of life. For the past 7 years this more than anything else has helped us all to cope. Christian was assessed by an occupational therapist for several weeks. His findings were that Christian was very lonely and isolated and that the best way forward was for Christian to employ a personal assistant (PA) who could help him to socialize. We can say in all honesty that he has done more in the past few years than he did in the 17 years leading up to employing a PA. Having a PA is helping Christian to live both independently and safely. It also helps us because we are sharing the burden of caring, which makes life much easier.

His current PA, Denise, has made significant improvements to his life. He now enjoys going to shows – often in London – shopping trips, breaks away and even holidays, something he has not enjoyed since he was a boy. Caring can be exhausting but these days I feel free to do things that I wasn't able to do before. We still have daily contact and provide support and a safe, inviting place for him to come whenever he likes, but I am not worrying 24 hours a day like I used to. He has employed five PAs, but I feel that only one of them has really suited Christian. Denise had first-hand experience of mental health problems and it was apparent from the start that, unlike his other PAs, she did not have to keep phoning me for advice on how to deal with problems that arose. Recovery is only possible if we can improve quality of life – medication is only one small part of the jigsaw.

There are many other essential elements that have helped our family's recovery and the lives of many other carers we have come to know. These include:

*Love* Mental illness strips people of their precious self-esteem. We believe that love and solid family support is the biggest mover in recovery.

*Compassion* Our son's illness was handled under a veil of secrecy, as if we didn't really exist. Had he been suffering from a physical condition we believe that we would have felt far more included. It's high time that mental health is given exactly the same level of understanding and compassion as physical illnesses. We need nurses who have been highly trained, like the Macmillan nurses. The suffering is so immense and yet people are still not being given respect for what they go through.

*Collaborative working partnerships* In recent years we have felt that practitioners have listened to us, but more importantly heard us. Carers have a wealth of experience that can be tapped into and used. We need to work with professionals as partners in care, both parties respecting each other for their individual but equally important expertise. Some professionals hide behind a smokescreen of patient confidentiality, even when the patient is happy for their carer to be involved in all aspects of their care. This is a big cause of 'high expressed emotion'. During the past 23 years Christian has had various nurses and social workers, some have been good and others let's just say not so good. His current social worker has been excellent and we both feel that she cares not just about Christian but about the family as a whole. She arranged for us to have a carers assessment with a view to accessing a personal budget as carers in our own right. We were asked what would help us to cope with caring; we discussed various options and came to the conclusion that respite breaks away from it all would be very beneficial. This has been set up this year as an ongoing arrangement. We feel that this is a really good example of collaborative partnerships. Working together as equal partners, respecting each other for our individual expertise and pooling it for the best possible results is imperative. Collaborative working only works well when the practitioner understands just how painful it is to be caught up in a situation where someone you love dearly suffers to the extent that Christian did and still does sometimes.

*Medication* We stress that it has to be the right medication, and it should be monitored and changed periodically if there is little or no improvement. People should be able to access clozapine as early as possible if other medicines do not work or cause intolerable side effects. Christian has side effects, but they are certainly more tolerable than the hell of his symptoms.

*Talking therapy*   Christian was lucky enough to have 3 years of a psychodynamic therapy that has given him an insight into his condition. Asking people to go through this journey without the benefit of talking therapy is like asking someone to climb a mountain without a compass, rope or light.

*Supported housing*   Christian has lived in his own flat for 10 years. Staff are there from 9.00 a.m. to 5.00 p.m. Monday to Friday but he relies less and less on their support, as the family and Denise provide most of it. Having said that, it is good to know they are there if ever he needs them. He has a self-contained one-bedroom flat and there is also shared accommodation and a dining room with a TV to encourage the residents to get together. Sometimes the mental health of the other residents impacts on the quality of Christian's life. We are trying to save enough money to buy him a private flat near to us. We feel he will be able to cope, providing he has our continued support and that of his PA.

*Part-time employment*   When Christian became well enough to work part-time we managed to help him secure a job in a warehouse, working 9 hours a week. After a couple of years he was made redundant, along with many others. We watched his mental health slowly deteriorate; the work had provided some much-needed structure to his life. I spoke to his social worker on many occasions, who seemed to think that we were just pushing him to go to work. I felt she refused to listen to us or accept that we knew that working had helped him so much. I work periodically for our local NHS trust delivering 'The Carer's Perspective', a programme aimed at helping new staff become more aware of the need to involve carers and families. I made an appointment with the chief executive, who offered Christian 6 hours a week in a local community hospital. He now works two afternoons a week doing administrative work, photocopying and addressing envelopes etc., which has helped him to socialize and also earn a wage. We feel that this has given him self-confidence and some much-needed structure. He likes to be able to say 'I go to work', he also enjoys being occupied. Boredom can cause many problems and having a reason to get up out of bed and get on with life has proved most beneficial. He has worked there successfully for the past 7 years; his manager and colleagues are understanding, supportive and flexible and work around him if he is having a bad day. They even allow him to come over to my house (which is opposite the hospital) for a cup of tea during his 15-minute tea break.

*Family therapy*   This was recommended by a consultant in the psychotherapy department of our local hospital. Christian and I attended monthly sessions for a year. We both learned a lot about our own behaviour and gradually started to become aware that we had become almost fused together. Family therapy slowly encouraged me to stop checking that he was OK and also made me realize that my behaviour was simply suggesting to him that he wasn't OK. It helped us to take a look at our own behaviour and address things accordingly. It has particularly helped me to stop 'over-caring'. For example, Christian would look to me for support but I was so scared of his condition that all he saw was my fear. I now react very differently, in a much calmer and measured way.

*Pets*   We've had four dogs during Christian's illness and now have a border terrier and an African grey parrot. As for the parrot, he's a great talker and no matter how down we may feel he can always manage to make us laugh.

*Attention to diet and physical exercise*   We encourage Chris to not have too many takeaway or ready meals. He stopped going swimming following the incident with the head teacher and police I mentioned earlier. It destroyed his confidence. Instead he walks a lot and regularly takes the dog for walks.

*Respite*   This is imperative to carers. As well as the personal budget Christian gets to employ his PA, we as carers are also given a budget for respite. We were assessed by Christian's social worker, who managed to get us a budget that was enough for a couple of weeks away in a bed and breakfast. We never had a holiday for 20 years, but now, even though the budget is reduced owing to cuts, we usually take two nights at a time and come back feeling refreshed and far more able to care for our son.

# Part 4
# PHYSICAL HEALTH IN SCHIZOPHRENIA

# 12

# Remember your physical health

Patients, carers, clinicians and researchers have been campaigning for a more holistic and integrated approach to physical and mental health care for many years. Surprisingly, it has only been in the past few years that policymakers have recognized that the physical health of people with schizophrenia and other mental illnesses has to be given the same priority as their mental health. GPs and mental health trusts now have targets to meet to improve both the mental and physical health of the people who use their services. This refocusing towards holistic health care delivery is central to the UK government's drive to reduce health inequalities, support people to make informed healthy choices and improve partnership working across services.

In this section of the book we aim to explain the types of physical health conditions people with schizophrenia may experience and their causes. In Chapter 15 we provide suggestions for managing and improving your physical health. But this book can provide only an introduction to looking after your physical health. For most of the topics we will discuss there are excellent articles on the main NHS Choices website <www.nhs.uk>. We strongly suggest that you follow up reading this book by going to the relevant websites.

# 13

## Physical health conditions in people with schizophrenia

People with schizophrenia experience exactly the same physical health conditions as those who do not experience mental health problems. They do, however, experience some physical health problems more frequently and in some cases more severely. We have known for many years that, on average, some (but not all) people who have a severe mental illness such as schizophrenia, bipolar disorder or long-term depression have a shorter life expectancy than people who are mentally healthy. Researchers have estimated that having a severe mental illness shortens a person's life by an average of 10–20 years. Now, before you get totally depressed by this shocking statistic, you need to know that this shortened life expectancy is mostly caused by *preventable* health conditions such as heart disease, diabetes, respiratory disease and some cancers.

The physical health problems we discuss here are not exhaustive but, as we mentioned at the beginning of the book, we believe that having access to the same information as health professionals is important for people with schizophrenia and their carers. Poor physical health is not inevitable. Being fully aware of potential problems gives you a true choice in whether or not to take on board the information and act to change things.

### Cardiovascular disease

Cardiovascular disease is the main cause of death for people living in the UK, accounting for 1 in 3 of all deaths, and also the leading cause of death in people with schizophrenia. It includes conditions such as heart disease, high blood pressure, high cholesterol and stroke. Getting older increases our risk of heart disease, as does having a parent with a heart condition. However, in more than 90 per cent of cases, the risk of having a first heart attack is related to nine things that are under our control (Yusuf *et al.* 2004):

- Abnormal ratio of fat in the blood
- Current smoking
- Diabetes
- High blood pressure
- Abdominal obesity
- Stress
- Low amount of fruit and vegetable in the daily diet
- Lack of exercise
- Excessive alcohol intake.

This list is presented in order of which factor has the most influence. The two most important risk factors are cigarette smoking and an abnormal ratio of fats in the blood (e.g. high cholesterol). Together, they predict two-thirds of the risk of heart attack. The impact of risk factors is the same in every ethnic group and in every region in the world. Having an awareness of these factors means we can choose whether or not to engage in these behaviours or take control to limit them.

## Respiratory disease

Respiratory conditions include chest infections, pneumonia, tuberculosis, asthma and chronic obstructive pulmonary disease (known as COPD). Until 50 years ago, respiratory diseases such as pneumonia and tuberculosis accounted for the majority of deaths among people with schizophrenia who lived in institutions. Such respiratory diseases are still more prevalent in people with schizophrenia than those in the general population who are mentally well, and are thought to result from high rates of smoking or passive smoking, poor diet, poverty and environmental factors.

## Cancers

One in four of all deaths in the UK are due to cancer. There are approximately 200 different types of cancer, each with different causes, such as viruses, a weakened immune system, poor diet and obesity. Tobacco use is the single most important risk factor for cancer. There are conflicting reports as to whether people with schizophrenia have lower, similar or higher rates of cancer than the general population. The confusion is mostly related to how, where and when research in this area of health care was carried out. One problem is that, compared with the general population, fewer people (particularly women) with schizophrenia attend routine cancer screening appointments, so are unlikely to be diagnosed. However, there seems to be fairly consistent evidence that people with schizophrenia have higher than expected rates of digestive and breast cancer, possibly related to obesity, alcohol use and medication-related changes in hormones.

## Nutritional and metabolic diseases

### Obesity

Obesity is a significant problem in the general population, as well as for people with schizophrenia and other serious mental illnesses. Approximately 60 per cent of adults in the UK are overweight or obese, and a similar proportion of people with schizophrenia, although a higher rate of upper body fat around the abdomen is more common in people with schizophrenia. Fat stored around the abdomen is a stronger risk factor for developing metabolic complications than overall body fat.

Weight gain in people with schizophrenia is mostly related to a sedentary lifestyle and poor diet. However, additional challenges faced by people with schizophrenia also play a part in obesity. Negative symptoms such as lack of motivation, and cognitive symptoms such as difficultly in planning ahead, along with the side effects of some medicines (weight gain and sedation) also need to be taken into consideration. The implications of obesity are an increased risk of developing diabetes, cardiovascular and respiratory disease and some cancers.

### Diabetes

There are two types of diabetes. Type 1 (previously known as insulin dependent) has a rapid onset and occurs when insulin-producing cells have been destroyed by the body's immune system. As a result, the body is unable to produce insulin and this leads to increased blood glucose (sugar) levels, which in turn can cause serious damage to other organs in the body. This often begins in childhood or adolescence. Type 2 diabetes (previously known as non-insulin dependent) has a much slower onset and often begins in the middle years of life. It develops when the body is unable to effectively use the insulin that is produced or when the body does not produce enough insulin to maintain a normal blood glucose level.

Diabetes in the general population often goes undiagnosed for many years – estimates suggest up to 12 years. The consequence of delayed diagnosis results in prolonged exposure to raised blood glucose and this can cause problems such as visual impairment and damage to the kidneys and nervous system.

Diabetes occurs in approximately 15 per cent of people with schizophrenia and possibly at an even higher rate in people with mood disorders; this compares with approximately 2–5 per cent in the general population. The causation of diabetes is influenced by a family history of diabetes, smoking, physical inactivity, poor diet and the effects of antipsychotic medication.

In recent years, health professionals and people with schizophrenia have become very concerned that antipsychotic medication causes diabetes. However, we have known for over a century that, even in people with schizophrenia who have never taken antipsychotic medication, diabetes occurs at a greater rate than in the general population. The most widely accepted explanation for this is that a genetic predisposition to insulin resistance is made worse by a poor diet, lack of activity, smoking and the effects of antipsychotic medication on weight and metabolism. To prevent and manage diabetes, we therefore need to pay attention to all these factors.

## Metabolic syndrome

This is the name for a group of risk factors that raises the risk for heart disease and other health problems, such as diabetes and stroke. There are number of definitions for metabolic syndrome, depending on which organization's guidelines you read. There seems to be general agreement among doctors that the major features of the syndrome are:

1  A large waistline (excess fat in the stomach area is a greater risk factor for heart disease than excess fat in other parts of the body).
2  High triglyceride level (triglycerides are a type of fat found in the blood).
3  Low HDL (high-density lipoprotein) cholesterol level (this is

sometimes called 'good' cholesterol because it helps remove cholesterol from the arteries. A low HDL cholesterol level raises your risk for heart disease).

4  High blood pressure.

5  High blood sugar.

You don't need to have all five conditions to be considered to have metabolic syndrome, only two or three of them.

## Viral diseases

People with schizophrenia have higher than expected rates of some long-term viral infections, such as HIV and hepatitis B and C. There is nothing about the actual disorder of schizophrenia that is directly related to increased rates of viral diseases; rather it has more to do with illicit drug use and health behaviours that a minority of people with schizophrenia sometimes engage in.

### HIV

HIV attacks the immune system and weakens the body's ability to fight infections and disease. A person with HIV is considered to have developed AIDS (acquired immune deficiency syndrome) when the immune system is so weak it can no longer fight life-threatening infections. The most common way of contracting HIV is by having unprotected sex with a person who has HIV (this includes vaginal, anal and oral sex). Other ways of contracting HIV include using a contaminated needle, syringe or other drug-injecting equipment, or transmission from mother to baby – before or during birth or by breastfeeding.

The number of people with schizophrenia (and other serious mental illnesses) who are HIV positive is higher than in the general population. So what might make people with schizophrenia more vulnerable to HIV? It is not schizophrenia as such, but the fact that people with schizophrenia who are sexually active are more likely to have unprotected sex for a whole range of reasons. Coercion to have unwanted sex is common in mental health settings, as is paying for or selling sex. Limited supportive social relationships, temporary accommodation and lack of privacy can all disrupt initiating and maintaining long-term relationships and lead to a tendency to have frequent and different partners.

Using a condom during sex is the best prevention against HIV and other diseases that are transmitted sexually. However, mental health facilities do not often make condoms easily (and anonymously) available to people who choose to have consensual sex during an inpatient stay or when they have ground or home leave or when living in the community. Offering routine testing for HIV status is becoming increasingly common in mental health settings and is important for improving the detection and treatment of HIV in people with mental health problems. HIV treatments have improved a great deal over recent years and HIV is now considered a manageable long-term condition.

## Hepatitis

Hepatitis is a term used to describe inflammation (swelling) of the liver. Again, this is preventable condition that if recognized early can be successfully treated. People are often unaware they have a form of hepatitis, as sometimes there are not any obvious symptoms or it is mistaken for flu. It can be caused by damaging the liver from using too much alcohol, or from our own autoimmune process (when the body attacks itself). However, infections are the most common cause of hepatitis and are caused by different strains of a virus (hepatitis A, B, C, D and E).

The hepatitis A infection is usually passed to others through preparing food, or through close contact with an infected person who has not washed their hands properly after going to the toilet. It is common in places where there is contaminated food and water. Most cases of hepatitis A in the UK are diagnosed in people returning home after travelling to a country where sanitation is poor. Flu-like symptoms, fever, tiredness, feeling sick, vomiting and diarrhoea, and an ache in the liver region (the upper part of the right side of the abdomen below your ribs) occur after a few weeks of being infected. This type of infection is unpleasant but is usually self-limiting and rarely leads to any long-term problems.

Hepatitis B and C are two other strains of the virus and are more common in people with schizophrenia and related serious mental illnesses compared with the general population. Hepatitis B is passed on either through unprotected sex or infected blood, usually from sharing needles or any injecting equipment (e.g. spoons, filters, water for injection). Sharing toothbrushes or razors with an infected person can also transmit the virus as it only takes a tiny drop of infected blood to enter the body to pass on the virus. It cannot be passed on during normal social contact, such as holding hands or sharing cups or other crockery. Often, people do not experience symptoms and the body can in effect 'treat' itself via the immune system and get rid of the virus. Some people may feel sick, have abdominal pains, fever, feel generally unwell and may become jaundiced (the skin looks yellow).

Hepatitis C is also passed on via infected blood but to a much lesser extent by other body fluids through unprotected sex. Like hepatitis B, it cannot be passed on during normal social contact. Again, there are usually no obvious symptoms, though infected people may feel continually tired. A small minority may experience long-term consequences of infection with hepatitis B and C viruses, such as cirrhosis (scarring) of the liver. This can lead to the liver not functioning properly. Because hepatitis B and C are increasingly seen in people with schizophrenia, routine screening is recommended for people who use mental health services. A simple blood test can detect hepatitis and treatment consists of a course of antiviral medicines.

## Osteoporosis

Osteoporosis is a condition where the bones become less dense and are more prone to breaking. Some people with schizophrenia are at higher risk of osteoporosis than people without the condition because of their health behaviours and because some antipsychotic medicines contribute to osteoporosis. Among these behaviours is smoking, which causes bone-damaging changes because it affects the absorption of calcium and kills bone-making cells. A diet that is low in calcium and a lack of exercise to strengthen the muscles to protect the bones also plays a part. What is more, bones get thinner as we age and when there is a fall in the levels of the hormone oestrogen – such as at the menopause. Finally, some medications, particularly the older antipsychotic medications, depot injections and some of the more recent medicines – risperidone, paliperidone and amisulpride – can indirectly affect bone density by increasing the levels of the hormone prolactin.

Mental health services are increasingly offering bone density scans to detect osteoporosis. Early detection, a review and a possible change of medication will reduce the risk of osteoporosis in people with schizophrenia. It is also important to be aware that one of the long-term benefits of stopping smoking is a reduction in the rate of bone loss as well as a reduced risk of hip fractures.

## Blood disorders

People who are prescribed clozapine will know only too well that it has a very small chance of causing problems with the white cells in the blood. The white cells (of which there are of a number of types) are important for the body's immune system and for fighting infection. Sometimes clozapine and, to a lesser extent, all the other antipsychotic medications can cause a reduction in white cells and make people more vulnerable to fighting infections.

People who are prescribed clozapine have their blood monitored very closely – weekly when they are first prescribed the medicine and eventually monthly. This is because the risk of harming the white cells reduces the longer the medicine is taken. But the risk never entirely goes away, which is why all the time someone is prescribed clozapine, blood tests will be needed. Symptoms of a very low white cell count may include fever, chills and infections, such as recurrent bacterial throat or skin infections, and constant body aches and pain. This condition is very rare and constant monitoring is a good way of preventing any serious conditions and means the drug can be altered or stopped.

Clozapine is licensed for people with schizophrenia who are described as treatment resistant (technically this means they have not responded to at least two other antipsychotics). As we mentioned in Chapter 7, it is considered to be the most effective medication for treating the symptoms of schizophrenia. When clozapine is suggested as a treatment option and the blood monitoring requirements are also explained it can seem overwhelming to patients and their families. As with any medication, the person taking it and their family must weigh up the good things and not so good things about each choice of medication. Clozapine is not the only medication that can affect the white cell count. Other antipsychotics can do this, as well as carbamazepine (a mood stabilizer) and some antidepressant medications.

## Anaemia

Anaemia develops when the blood lacks enough healthy red blood cells (and therefore the haemoglobin within). If you have too few red blood cells, or they are abnormal, the cells in your body will not get enough oxygen. There are many types of anaemia and many different causes, such as reduced production of red cells, a lack of minerals (e.g. iron) and vitamins (e.g. vitamin B12) needed for red blood cells to work properly, and long-term use of drugs such as aspirin or ibuprofen.

Psychiatric symptoms have long been attributed to vitamin B12 deficiency and, more recently, folate deficiency (vitamin B9). People with schizophrenia have been found to have lower levels of these than healthy people. Vitamin B12 and folate work together to help the body produce red blood cells. They also have several other important functions, such as keeping the nervous system healthy. Symptoms of iron or vitamin B12 deficiency include tiredness, lethargy (lack of energy), shortness of breath, headaches and tinnitus (ringing in your ears). Deficiencies have also been associated with negative symptoms and neurological symptoms such as confusion and poor memory.

## Oral health

Poor oral health is linked to conditions such as coronary heart disease and stroke. Bacteria from our mouths can enter the bloodstream from bleeding gums; once bacteria get into the bloodstream they can trigger clotting inside blood vessels, increasing the risk of heart attacks and stroke.

People with a serious mental illness such as schizophrenia have higher rates of tooth decay and tooth loss compared with mentally healthy people. This may be because they face additional challenges of maintaining good oral hygiene. Poor oral health is caused by a number of factors, such as smoking (which causes the gums and bone to recede as well as tooth loss), poor diet (e.g. food and drink with high sugar content) and some antipsychotic medicines (which reduce the flow of saliva in the mouth, resulting in dry mouth).

Easy access to dental care, regardless of whether or not someone has a mental health problem, is a public health concern in the UK and other areas of the world, and can be a major barrier to maintaining good oral health.

As we mentioned earlier in this chapter, this is not a complete list of physical health problems that people with schizophrenia may encounter. It is vital that you consult a health professional if you are concerned about any symptoms you are experiencing.

# 14

# Reasons for poor physical health

As you can see from Chapter 13, many physical health problems are caused by the interaction of several factors – rarely by just one. A number of reasons have been suggested for the association between severe mental illness and poor physical health, including a lack of integration of care between primary (GP) and secondary care (mental health trusts), the side effects of antipsychotic medications and the consequences of health behaviours such as smoking and diet.

## Lack of integration between primary and secondary care

Although there has been an improvement in the detection and treatment of physical health problems in people with schizophrenia in recent years, unfortunately this is not a consistent experience for all. It is condemnable that poor access to and provision of health services contribute to poor health outcomes in people with schizophrenia.

Some people still fall into the gap that exists between primary and secondary care. When you are in the midst of experiencing mental health problems it is sometimes confusing to work out who you need to consult if you develop a physical health problem. People with schizophrenia report that their physical health conditions are often overlooked or are put down to having a mental health condition. This may have something to do with the fact that, until fairly recently, mental health staff, although willing to be more involved in physical health care, had very little training in how to look after the physical health care needs of people with a mental illness, and that staff who work in GP practices had very little training in how to look after the mental health care needs of their patients with a physical health condition. There has also been a lack of implementation into routine mental health services of interventions that we know to work in general care settings (such as smoking cessation treatment).

## Physical effects of antipsychotic medication

We discussed in Chapter 7 some of the side effects of antipsychotic medication and what causes them. Weight gain, sedation, raised glucose levels, abnormal levels of fat in the blood and raised levels of the hormone prolactin all compromise the health of people with schizophrenia. Patients, carers and prescribers have to constantly weigh up the benefits and costs of each medication. Many of the health consequences of medication can be prevented or minimized through careful monitoring and health promotion interventions at the beginning of antipsychotic treatment.

## Illness-related factors

We also need to take into account the effect of severe mental illness on help-seeking behaviour. It has been suggested that people with schizophrenia are less likely to spontaneously report physical symptoms and may be unaware of physical problems because of the cognitive deficits associated with their schizophrenia. Non-adherence to prescribed medication is common in people prescribed medication for any long-term condition, and has a negative effect on physical and mental health outcomes.

There are also socio-economic consequences of having a mental health disorder, such as poverty, poor housing, reduced social networks, lack of employment and meaningful occupation opportunities, and social stigma, all of which impact on the physical health and the physical health behaviours of people with schizophrenia.

## Health behaviours

Increased rates of disease and death in people with schizophrenia are also caused by high rates of smoking, poor diet, lack of exercise, substance use and unsafe sexual practices. These behaviours are often referred to by health professionals as 'lifestyle choices'. Patients, however, would probably argue that these are not choices at all, but the physical, psychological, social and environmental consequences of having a severe mental illness and the treatments prescribed for them. Let's look at these behaviours in a bit more detail.

## Smoking

People with a mental health problem such as schizophrenia, or even bipolar disorder, depression and anxiety, are more likely to smoke. About 60 per cent of people with schizophrenia smoke, and adults with mental health problems, including those who misuse alcohol or drugs, smoke 42 per cent of all the tobacco used in England (McManus *et al.* 2010). In the general UK population, about 20 per cent of people smoke.

If you are a smoker you are more likely to have poor general health; smoking is one of the main reasons why people with a mental illness tend to die younger than people who are mentally well. Smoking is the largest preventable cause of death in the UK (and the rest of the world) and is responsible for an average reduction in life expectancy of 10 years. People with schizophrenia are more likely to be heavier smokers and more nicotine dependant than smokers in the general population, and are less likely to be offered smoking cessation support.

There are many reasons why people with schizophrenia may have such high rates of smoking. People who smoke, regardless of whether they have a mental health problem, say they smoke to help them manage the stress of day-to-day living. Smoking is perceived to be calming, relaxing and mood enhancing. Indeed, it can be those things! However, the reason why a smoker comes to experience smoking as stress relieving needs to be understood. Rarely does anyone start smoking because they think it will be a good way to deal with stress. We usually start smoking for social reasons – because we see our friends and family smoking, it seems a cool thing to do, and we think it helps us look and feel older. We tell ourselves that we can stop when we want to but before we know it we are smoking every day, all day.

You inhale approximately 4,000 chemicals from a single cigarette, 60 of which are known to cause cancer. It is mostly the nicotine that keeps you smoking. Inhaling smoke from tobacco is a highly efficient method of absorbing nicotine into the bloodstream and it only takes a few seconds for it to reach the brain. There, it stimulates the release of dopamine as well as other neurotransmitters such as serotonin and adrenaline.

However, the nicotine from a cigarette does not stay in the body for very long and as your levels start to drop you start to experience withdrawal symptoms, such as nicotine craving, irritability, anxiety, restlessness, low mood and impaired concentration. To prevent these awful feelings, the easiest and quickest thing to do is have another cigarette. Regulating your nicotine levels every 30–60 minutes will prevent these withdrawal symptoms. If you leave it any longer you will start feeling grumpy and maybe a bit low in mood and anxious. If you have nothing to distract you it will get to the point where you can't think of anything else other than having a cigarette. A reasonable explanation for why smokers (those with and without a mental illness) perceive cigarettes to be calming and stress relieving is that regular smoking stops the onset of nicotine withdrawal symptoms; the apparent relaxant effect of smoking only reflects the reversal of the tension and irritability that develops as the nicotine level in your brain reduces.

Smokers, carers and mental health clinicians often exaggerate the perceived benefits of smoking. They often attribute improved mood and reduced anxiety to the effects of smoking rather than the reality that smoking simply medicates the effects of nicotine withdrawal that occur several times throughout the day. They also worry that stopping smoking will cause their mental health to deteriorate. If you choose to stop smoking, providing you get support and use nicotine replacement therapy or other medicines approved to help people stop smoking, then your mental health will not deteriorate. In fact, stopping smoking can improve your mental health.

If you take a group of people who smoke, a group who are ex-smokers and a group who have never smoked and test their levels of stress, anxiety or their symptoms such as voices, the current smokers will have the highest levels of mental health symptoms and the ex-smokers will have fewer symptoms than the smokers. The people with the lowest levels of stress and mental health symptoms will be the group who have never smoked.

Simply knowing that smoking is a major cause of feeling stressed in the first place, rather than the only way to relieve stress, can be a helpful starting point for understanding the physical reason why people smoke. However, the relationship between smoking and schizophrenia is a little more complicated. Staying on the subject of nicotine withdrawal symptoms, researchers have found that compared with smokers without a mental illness, people with schizophrenia may be more sensitive to the effects of abruptly stopping smoking; they experience nicotine withdrawal symptoms earlier and more intensely shortly after smoking a cigarette than mentally well smokers who have similar levels of dependence and similar smoking patterns. It appears that the ability to tolerate the gaps between smoking a cigarette may be limited owing to the additional internal and external challenges of having a mental illness.

Smoking has been an accepted and expected part of the culture of psychiatry for many years and many people with a mental illness report a lack of encouragement from mental health professionals to stop smoking. They also report that a number of mental health staff use cigarettes to help develop a relationship with them, to motivate, punish and reward behaviour change, and to fill time.

Inpatient wards are notorious for the high level of boredom experienced by patients. Although all wards offer some occupational therapy, this generally amounts to 2 hours twice a day, with little else apart from the TV to offer any distraction. Boredom is an obvious factor in increasing the frequency of smoking; patients often say there is nothing else to do *but* smoke!

Smoking is often viewed as a shared experience and thus reduces the feeling of isolation. It provides opportunities to make friends, interact and connect with others. Patients are often afraid of losing this perceived benefit, despite the negative impact of smoking; they see it as one of the few things they can control in their lives. With good mental health care there should be alternative and healthier solutions offered to people to gain a sense of control in their lives.

Smoking bans have been widely implemented throughout the UK, Europe, Australia and North America to protect the health of non-smokers. Since 2008, patients admitted to a mental health unit in the UK have not been able to smoke indoors and some hospitals have banned or restricted smoking in the hospital grounds. Many patients who smoke, as well as their carers and clinicians, have complained that being prevented from smoking while in hospital is an infringement of their rights. Banning smoking certainly poses an ethical and moral dilemma. However, smoking bans are not simply restricted to mental health settings but apply to all enclosed places where people work and the public and patients have access. To have special exemptions in place to allow smoking for people who are receiving hospital treatment for a mental illness does little to support the argument for equality for people with mental health problems.

We cannot strive to bring to an end to the stigma and discrimination that people with a mental illness face in all aspects of life while passively accepting the excessive rates of smoking and the resultant disproportionate illness and premature death experienced as a result.

## Diet and exercise

The physical health consequences of a poor diet include coronary heart disease, diabetes, obesity, some cancers, osteoporosis and tooth decay. Although the overall diet of the British public has improved in the past 20 years, the consumption of fruit, vegetables, oily fish, wholegrain products and fibre is still below the recommended levels and most of the adult population consumes more than the recommended maximum 6 g of salt a day. It is therefore not at all surprising that some people with schizophrenia also have a diet that does not meet health recommendations.

We know from surveys of people with schizophrenia that their intake of fruit and vegetables is lower and that they consume more calories than the general population; this does not just occur in people living at home but can also be seen during inpatient admissions. A healthy, balanced diet is also important for maintaining good mental health. Poor mental health outcomes in schizophrenia are associated with a diet high in saturated fat and refined sugar, whereas consumption of fish and seafood, particularly omega-3 fatty acids, is associated with better outcomes.

The WHO identifies poor diet and physical inactivity as one of the leading causes of death in developed countries. People who have a sedentary lifestyle, do not participate in moderate or vigorous physical activity and watch more than 4 hours of television a day are more prone to obesity and cardiovascular disease risk factors. People with schizophrenia and bipolar disorder are less physically active than the general population and are less likely to be encouraged to exercise by health workers. In a cross-sectional survey of 120 people with a mental illness, fatigue, mental health symptoms and lack of confidence were reported as the main barriers to regular exercise. Over half the respondents were positive about the benefits of exercise and said they were motivated to be more active (Ussher et al. 2007).

## Substance use

People who have schizophrenia and drink alcohol excessively or use illicit drugs face a greater challenge in maintaining their physical health, as the effects of substance use compound the physical health issues associated with schizophrenia. Long-term alcohol abuse results in cardiovascular and liver disease, as well as immune and gastrointestinal disorders. Stimulants such as cocaine increase the heart rate and blood pressure, which in turn increase the oxygen demand on the heart. Excessive alcohol intake increases the risk of cancers of the mouth, throat, oesophagus, colon and breast.

Unlike cigarette smoking, the effect of cannabis on the lungs has been poorly understood until recently. Some studies suggest that it is associated with obstructive lung disease, which seems to occur earlier in cannabis smokers than in tobacco smokers. This may be due to cannabis smokers inhaling more and holding their breath four times longer than cigarette smokers, which increases the concentration and lung deposits from the smoke and leads to greater and more rapid lung destruction. Many people with schizophrenia smoke tobacco and cannabis together, which may well increase the risk of developing respiratory symptoms even further.

Most of the physical health problems we have discussed in the book are due to preventable conditions, meaning preventable by health services and health professionals and preventable by people with schizophrenia and their families. It also means preventable from a societal perspective – by better regulation of the food industry, creating better access to transport, ensuring that people with mental health problems have access to adequate housing and employment etc. Achieving optimal physical health needs a collaborative effort between all parties and each person concerned needs to know who is doing what, why, when and how.

Improvements are being made within the health service to be better at preventing physical health problems and at detecting them early and treating them effectively. However, the part of the country you live in still dictates the type and quality of care you receive, not just for mental health problems, but for any type of health care. What we aim to do in Chapter 16 is make you aware of the physical health checks and treatment people with schizophrenia should be offered and offer suggestions for improving your health.

# 15

# Taking control of health issues

## Weight

### Knowing if you are a healthy weight

Being a healthy weight will help control your blood pressure and blood glucose levels, and helps reduce the risk of heart disease and diabetes. It is not unusual for weight to rapidly increase when you first start taking antipsychotic medication. Preventing weight gain in the first place is easier than losing weight once you have put it on. As well as regular weighing, another way to check if you are overweight is by calculating your body mass index (BMI). You can calculate your own BMI; you need to measure your height in metres and your weight in kilograms. Then divide your weight by your height. Then divide the number you arrive at by your height again. There are many online tools that can do the calculations for you, such as: <www.nhs.uk/tools/pages/healthyweightcalculator.aspx?WT.mc_id=101007>.

A normal BMI is 18.5 to 24.9. A BMI of less than 18.5 means you are underweight and may need to put on weight. A BMI of 24.9 or over means you are overweight, and over 30 means you are classed as obese. In recent years experts have suggested that measuring waist circumference (i.e. abdominal obesity) may be a more valid and reliable predictor of the risk of diabetes and cardiovascular disease than measuring overall obesity. To accurately measure the circumference of your waist, wrap the tape measure around your waist so it crosses your belly button. Guidelines for a healthy waist size differ depending on ethnicity. As a guide, men with a waist measurement of more than 94 cm and women with a measurement more than 80 cm are more likely to develop type 2 diabetes and heart problems (compared with having fat around the bottom or thighs).

## Eating a healthy diet

For a diet to be considered healthy, we need to balance the amount of food we eat with how active we are, and also eat a range of foods. Men need around 2,500 calories a day to keep their weight stable whereas women need around 2,000. However, people need fewer calories than this if they are not very active and spend most of their day sitting down. Nowadays, a great deal of information is available about the type of foods we should eat more of and those we should eat less of. We often hear contradictory messages about what is good for us. For example, one minute we hear that drinking coffee is good for us, the next that we should avoid it. The Department of Health is always reviewing what the best evidence is for staying healthy.

Regarding our diet, the current recommendation is that it should mostly be made up of fruit, vegetables and starchy foods such as wholegrain rice and pasta or potatoes. The rest should consist of proteins such as meat, fish or beans as well as a small amount of dairy (e.g. milk, eggs and cheese). Foods that contain sugar and fat, such as cakes and biscuits, should only make up a very small amount of our diet. Sometimes people are not sure where to start with healthy eating and may need a bit of guidance. There will be professionals in mental health teams, such as occupational therapists, who are a good source of information and practical advice. People often worry that eating healthily is expensive, whereas the opposite is actually true. For example, the cost of a single banana is 2–3 times less than a bar of chocolate and will satisfy your hunger for longer.

### Fruit and vegetables

For many years now we have been encouraged to eat at least 5 portions of fruit and vegetables every day. This is based on advice from the WHO, which recommends eating a minimum of 400 g of fruit and vegetables a day to lower the risk of serious health problems such as heart disease, stroke, type 2 diabetes and obesity. Fruit and vegetables contain fibre, vitamins and minerals and have very few calories.

Many people struggle to eat this amount every day and it does take some effort and persistence if you are not used to it. Try tinned or frozen varieties as well, and unsweetened fruit juices or smoothies, bearing in mind that these only count as one portion because they have less fibre than the whole fruit. A portion is about 80 g or the size of your fist. So an apple or an orange is one portion, as is a handful of grapes, a large carrot or three tablespoons of peas. The way we cook food affects its nutrient content. Vegetables keep more of their vitamins and minerals if you lightly steam or bake them instead of boiling or frying them.

## Starchy foods

Potatoes, bread, rice, pasta and cereals are all types of starchy foods and provide us with energy; they are our main source of carbo-hydrates. There has been a great deal of misinformation about carbohydrates over recent years, mostly generated by celebrities who adopt low-carbohydrate diets as a way to lose weight rapidly (and unhealthily). These types of foods are not fattening if eaten in moderation – gram for gram they contain less than half the calories of fat.

Starchy foods also contain fibre, calcium, iron and B vitamins. Fibre is particularly important to help keep our bowels healthy. It also helps us to feel full, which means we are less likely to eat too much. Wholegrain and wholemeal varieties of starchy foods have more fibre and vitamins than processed grains (e.g. wholemeal bread compared with white bread) and potatoes with their skins on have more fibre than peeled potatoes. Starchy foods can be filling, nutritious and cheap; they become unhealthy when we smother them in foods that contain fat and sugars – putting sugar on cereals, covering a jacket potato in butter.

## Proteins from meat, fish and eggs

We need protein to help the body repair itself. The latest guidance from the Department of Health is that we should try and keep the amount of meat we eat to about 70 g a day (about two slices).

Some meats are high in fat, particularly saturated fat, which can raise cholesterol levels in the blood, thus raising your risk of heart disease. Too much red meat and processed meats like bacon and sausages also increase the risk of bowel cancer. The saturated fat from meat can be minimized by the way we prepare it before cooking and how we cook it. Trimming off all visible fat and grilling rather than frying is healthier. For example, fried chicken in breadcrumbs contains nearly six times as much fat as chicken grilled without the skin.

Fish on the other hand is very low in fat, and oily fish such salmon and mackerel are a good source of omega-3 fatty acids, which may prevent heart disease. Eggs are a good source of protein and full of vitamins. Pulses such as beans and lentils are also a good source of protein, as well as fibre, vitamins and minerals such as iron. They can be eaten as an alternative or in addition to meat. Milk, cheese and yoghurts are good sources of protein and calcium, provided they are low-fat varieties.

### Fats

We also need fat in our diet as well as carbohydrates and proteins. Fat provides energy and allows the body to absorb some necessary nutrients, such as vitamins A, D and E. There are two main types of fat found in food: unsaturated and saturated. Unsaturated fats are considered to be the more healthy. Unsaturated fats come from some plants and nuts, for example olive oil, sunflower oil and avocados. Other healthy fats come from oily fish. The unhealthy (saturated) fats come from animal products. Eating a diet high in saturated fat can cause the level of cholesterol in your blood to build up over time. Raised cholesterol increases your risk of heart disease. Foods high in saturated fat include meat, butter, hard cheese, pies, biscuits, cakes and pastries. It's important to eat the healthy types of fat and minimize the unhealthy ones.

It's very important to pay attention to both diet and exercise, as a healthy diet and being physically active have been linked with better mental health. Get as much support as you can on these topics from professionals to help with this.

### Maintaining a healthy weight

To maintain a healthy weight you need to balance the calories from the food and drink you consume with the amount of calories you burn through being active. To lose weight in a healthy way you need to use up more calories than you eat, such as by being more active. Losing weight slowly and steadily is much healthier than going on a crash diet. Skipping meals is not a helpful way to lose weight either – it only makes snacking on cakes, biscuits and sweets more tempting. Planning meals a day or two in advance instead of making decisions on a moment-to-moment basis gives you more control over what you eat.

## Getting enough exercise

A number of studies have demonstrated the positive benefits of exercise on both physical and mental health. To stay healthy or to improve health we need to do two types of physical activity each week: aerobic and muscle-strengthening activity. Aerobic activities improve cardiovascular health and include brisk walking, cycling, jogging, swimming and dancing, anything that gets your heart rate up and gets you out of breath. Muscle-strengthening exercises improve balance, muscle tone and bone health, increase the rate at which the body burns calories and can be achieved by climbing stairs, carrying shopping, walking uphill, gardening, yoga or t'ai chi. The latest guidelines from the Department of Health suggest we should do at least 150 minutes (2 hours and 30 minutes) of moderate intensity aerobic activity each week and some muscle-strengthening activities at least twice a week. Moderate intensity means working hard enough to be breathing more heavily than normal, becoming slightly warmer, but still be able to talk.

We need to get creative about how we can incorporate exercise into our daily routine without much effort or disruption – for example, exercising for two 10-minute intervals each day might be initially more achievable than half an hour at a time on 5 days of the week. Most mental health trusts now employ exercise trainers. These are a valuable source of support. Trainers can assess your current level of fitness and work out an individual exercise programme to suit your fitness needs and confidence. Personal exercise trainers should be accessible during both inpatient stays and when in the community. If you prefer to go to your local gym, you can often get discounted rates of membership with a referral from your GP.

## Managing your medication

Negotiate a change of medication if you think yours is contributing to your weight gain. As we discussed in Chapter 7, weight gain is greatest for clozapine and olanzapine, while quetiapine and risperidone have an intermediate risk. Amisulpride and aripiprazole have little effect on weight. For people who receive treatment for their first episode of psychosis, all antipsychotics are likely to cause weight gain. Other medicines such as mood stabilizers (e.g. lithium and sodium valproate) and some antidepressants (e.g. mirtazapine) can also cause weight gain.

## Taking control of blood pressure

As we have noted in Chapter 13, people with schizophrenia are at greater risk of cardiovascular illness and early death, both of which are mostly preventable. An important risk factor for heart disease and stroke is raised blood pressure, and there is a great deal you can do to ensure that your blood pressure remains within normal limits.

When your heart beats it pumps blood round your body, and as the blood moves it pushes against the sides of the blood vessels. The strength of this pushing is your blood pressure. If your blood pressure is too high it puts extra strain on the heart and this may lead to heart attacks and strokes.

Blood pressure is measured in millimetres of mercury (mmHg). Ideally, our blood pressure should be lower than 120/80 mmHg. The first (or top) number is called the systolic blood pressure. It is the highest level your blood pressure reaches when your heart beats. The second (or bottom) number is called the diastolic blood pressure and is the lowest level your blood pressure reaches as your heart relaxes between beats. High blood pressure is diagnosed if readings on a number of separate occasions consistently show your blood pressure is 140/90 mmHg or higher. If you have diabetes or another condition that affects the circulation then you should aim to get your blood pressure below 130/80 mmHg. It's preferable to prevent high blood pressure in the first place by making healthy choices about your behaviour relating to diet, exercise and smoking. You don't have to wait until you have high blood pressure to make healthy lifestyle changes. However, if you are diagnosed with high blood pressure there is much you can do to lower it. The more you can reduce your blood pressure, the lower your risk of a heart attack or stroke will be. There a number of changes you can make to lower your blood pressure.

## Lifestyle changes

Eating more fruit and vegetables, maintaining a healthy weight, getting physically active and stopping smoking will all lower your blood pressure. As will eating less salt. Salt makes the body retain water, so if you eat too much the extra water stored in your body raises your blood pressure. An adult should eat no more than 6 g of salt a day. It's difficult to know how much salt you are eating unless you read food labels. Foods such as bread, ketchup, stock cubes and ready meals are usually high in salt. Not adding salt to meals will help to reduce your intake and substituting salt with other flavourings such as herbs and spices is another healthy option.

## Medication for high blood pressure

We strongly suggest that you look at the articles on the NHS Choices website: <www.nhs.uk/conditions/Blood-pressure-(high)/Pages/Introduction.aspx>. Medication to lower blood pressure is recommended for people who have persistent blood pressure readings over 140/90 mmHg. People with other cardiovascular risk factors such as diabetes should be offered treatment if they have persistent blood pressure over 130/85 mmHg. Just as with any other medication, this needs to be taken consistently for as long as it is prescribed, with regular blood pressure checkups. Machines that can be used at home can be bought at your local pharmacy and are a useful way of keeping a check on your day-to-day health.

## Taking control of cholesterol levels

Cholesterol is a type of fat. The body needs cholesterol to help make certain vitamins and hormones and can make enough of its own. We also get extra cholesterol from some of the foods we eat (dietary cholesterol) but this cholesterol is not the major cause of high cholesterol levels in the body. It is eating too much food with a high saturated fat content, such as meat and cheese, that is the main cause of a high cholesterol level, which can lead to serious problems like heart disease. It's not just eating too much saturated fat that causes high cholesterol – there are contributing factors. Among these is smoking, which lowers the amount of 'good' HDL cholesterol (see Chapter 13), as does having diabetes or an underactive thyroid (hypothyroidism).

People on antipsychotic medication need to have a blood test about 3 months after starting treatment and then at least every year to check their cholesterol levels. Ways to prevent or reduce a high cholesterol level are eating a healthy diet, regular exercise and stopping smoking. There are also medications called statins that can be prescribed by your GP if your cholesterol is not reducing from diet and exercise alone. It is common for cholesterol monitoring to be overlooked. It can be helpful for you or your family to prompt a health professional such as your GP or care coordinator to carry out these checks, and to keep your own record of the results.

## Taking control of glucose (blood sugar) levels

Glucose monitoring is not only necessary for people with diabetes. If you do have diabetes you will need to monitor your levels at least twice a day using test strips that you can get on prescription from your GP. However, everyone taking an antipsychotic medicine should have their blood tested every 6–12 months to assess their glucose levels. Again, glucose monitoring can be overlooked by health professionals so don't be hesitant about prompting them to check it regularly.

As we mentioned in Chapter 13, high blood glucose and diabetes are more common in people with schizophrenia, so it is important that you and your carers watch out for the signs and symptoms. These can include passing urine more often than usual, especially at night, feeling more thirsty than usual, extreme tiredness, losing weight without trying, blurred vision, slow healing of cuts and wounds, genital itching and regular episodes of thrush. Report any of these symptoms to your GP or care coordinator. Again, as with all areas of health, diet, exercise and stopping smoking will improve glucose control. Every GP practice will have access to nurses who specialize in the prevention and management of diabetes; they can be a great source of support and information so make sure you see them if you need to.

## Taking control of smoking

Stopping smoking is one of the best things you can do to improve your overall heath. But many smokers (with or without a mental health problem) struggle to give up, or manage to give up and then go back to smoking. It is easier to take control of your smoking if you have support. Getting support from an NHS Stop Smoking Service (there are about 150 in the UK) quadruples the chance of successfully stopping compared with having no support. The service offers free help, consisting of psychological support and free prescriptions for medicines to help minimize nicotine withdrawal symptoms. Increasingly, mental health professionals are receiving training to provide specialist advice to help people with mental health problems quit. In the future it is likely that providing smoking cessation support to people with mental health problems will become routine practice within mental health settings.

Smoking cessation treatment can be delivered either in a group or on a one-to-one basis. You are given a choice of gradually reducing the number of cigarettes you smoke before quitting or support to abruptly quit. One of the main reasons it is difficult to stop is because of nicotine withdrawal symptoms (e.g. irritability, anxiety and low mood). As well as having psychological support, having medicine to minimize these symptoms increases your chances of quitting and makes the whole process more bearable. Nicotine replacement therapy is the most commonly used medicine. It works best if you have two types together (e.g. patches and gum) and use it for about 3 months. There are other effective types of medication specifically for stopping smoking in the form of tablets that your GP can prescribe. Smoking cessation treatment that is effective for smokers in the general population can be just as effective for people with schizophrenia who smoke, providing the maximum amount of nicotine replacement is used and taken for as long as needed.

## Cancer screening checkups

There are a number of cancer screening programmes for which everyone is eligible; however, the uptake of cancer screening services is generally poor for people with schizophrenia. Women between the ages of 25 and 64 are eligible for a free cervical screening test every 3–5 years. The NHS breast screening programme provides free breast screening every 3 years for all women aged 50 to 70. The most recent screening programme to be introduced in the UK is for bowel cancer. This offers screening every 2 years to all men and women aged 60 to 69. Early detection of cancer improves your prognosis. When you become eligible for any cancer screening, your GP will automatically send you a letter inviting you to attend the GP practice or local hospital. It is very important not to ignore these letters. If you are uncertain or reluctant to attend, speak to your GP or mental health team, who will be able to provide you with information and help in finding someone to accompany you to the appointment.

You can also keep a check on your own health by self-examination. You can pick up a leaflet from your GP surgery or check online about breast and testicular self-examination; these resources provide simple instructions about what to feel and look for and what to discuss with your GP.

## Vaccinations

People over the age of 65 and those who are susceptible to complications of flu, such as people with respiratory diseases or diabetes, are encouraged to have a flu vaccination every year. Each year, the viruses that are most likely to cause flu are identified in advance and vaccines are made to increase immunity against them. Because strains of the flu virus change often, it is necessary to have a new flu jab every year. Recently, many mental health trusts in the UK have also started to offer flu jabs in the winter months, when flu can spread quickly in hospitals. There are several myths about the flu jab, such as having it actually gives you flu. Your GP surgery or health professional can give you accurate information about this.

Another vaccination that people may want to consider is that for hepatitis B. This should be considered by people who have liver disease, those who inject drugs or have a partner who injects drugs and people who frequently change sexual partners. Three injections over the course of 6 months are needed and provide immunity for around 5 years.

## Dental checkups and optician appointments

Looking after the health of your teeth, gums and eyes is important, particularly as some medicines may cause a dry mouth and blurred vision. People on income support can get free dental checkups and treatment. If you are over 60, have diabetes or are on income support you can get a free eye test every year. Again, it might feel like a bit of effort to organize this but it is worth preventing problems or detecting them early.

## Contraception and safe sex

Advice on sexual health can be found from a variety of places, such as your GP, sexual health clinics, family planning or contraception clinics. There is a huge amount of information you can access online that clearly and simply explains all aspects of sexual health, such as at <www.nhs.uk/livewell/sexualhealthtopics>. There are also online tools to assess how safe your sex life is: <www.nhs.uk/Tools/Pages/Safesextool.aspx>.

People can feel a bit embarrassed talking about their sexual health needs and end up never raising the issue. They are then left wondering whether some of the issues they are experiencing are normal or are a cause for concern. Don't let embarrassment get in the way of this important aspect of your health. There are many different methods of contraception and every GP practice will have a doctor or nurse who has special training in this area who can discuss your particular needs or refer you to another professional. They can also advise about the prevention of sexually transmitted diseases and provide access to free condoms.

Sexual health clinics are a valuable source of support and can also provide advice about any worries you may have about any part of your sex life. There are many medicines (e.g. antipsychotics, antidepressants and treatments for high blood pressure) that can make you feel like not having sex or reduce the pleasure you might get from sex. Raising your concerns will enable health professionals to alter your medication or help you to get the best support.

## Managing appointments with health professionals

Your first port of call for any health problem is your GP. Some people do not have a GP or prefer to speak to their mental health team. This is absolutely fine, though if you need referring to a specialist then your GP is usually the person who will arrange this. Making an appointment to see a GP requires some skill nowadays.

The first thing you have to do is negotiate your way past the receptionist and the systems in place to book an appointment. Anyone
who has tried to book a GP appointment in the UK will know that
these systems are not designed around people who have mental
health problems – some would say they are not designed around
patients at all!

Often you are required to phone early in the morning to request
an appointment for that day. If all the appointments have gone
then you can request an emergency appointment or book for
another day. If you do manage to see the doctor then the appointment will last approximately 5 minutes, just enough time to
address one problem. If you have these experiences then there are
ways to cope with the barriers.

Although you cannot always predict when you are going to be ill,
you can reliably predict that you will need regular ongoing contact
with your GP practice as well as your mental health team. So plan
ahead. Book an appointment in advance. When you see your GP
explain any difficulties you have in seeing them regularly and
request a regular appointment with him or her. Ask if you can book
these appointments in advance, rather than trying to get one on
the actual day. Also, ask for a double appointment – two appointment slots back to back – so that you have sufficient time to discuss
your problems. If you struggle to get out of bed, request an appointment for later in the day, to maximize the chance of making it.

Before each appointment, write down the things you want to
discuss (we gave an example of this when we discussed medication
in Chapter 7). If you feel awkward about speaking to the doctor
then take a friend or family member with you. It is much better to
plan ahead than try and deal with a crisis. For example, if you are
disorganized about collecting repeat prescriptions, have ran out of
medication, are frantically trying to get to see a GP and then the
receptionist tells you there are no appointments available, you are
understandably going to be stressed! Arranging a regular 3-monthly
appointment that coincides with getting a repeat prescription may
be more helpful. Undoubtedly, crises and emergency situations will
crop up from time to time. Each GP and mental health service will
have their own procedures for responding to crises; make sure you
know what these procedures are. Many parts of the country now
have easily accessible walk-in clinics that you can turn up to without
an appointment.

# Conclusion

The Schizophrenia Commission called schizophrenia the 'abandoned illness'. In our opinion this epithet is most descriptive and is by no means a dramatization of the state of care and treatment for this illness in the UK today.

Twenty years ago the government of the day made cancer, heart disease and mental illness its key priorities. Today, services for people with cancer are much improved and the progress in training heart surgeons and providing the best treatments for a number of cardiac conditions has been dramatic. But sadly, services for those with mental illness, and schizophrenia in particular, remain poor, as demonstrated by the recent National Audit, although there are some exceptions in a small number of NHS trusts around the country. We hope that in this short book we have shown that there is a great deal that could be done to improve the lot of people with schizophrenia by improving services and getting effective interventions to all those in need. This means that professionals must improve their practice; however, this can only be achieved with more equitable funding for mental health services.

Perhaps more importantly, we sincerely believe that there is a great deal that people with schizophrenia and their families can do for themselves. Our book is an attempt to provide the necessary knowledge and advice, and we hope that it will be widely read. Even now, in writing this conclusion, we realize that we may have missed some topics or given some topics insufficient attention. For these shortcomings we apologize. We believe, however, that we have pointed to the most important topics – treatments and physical health. We say this bearing in mind the fact that medications remain the mainstay of treatment and that, in our opinion, inadequate attention to physical health leads to the needless waste of years of life. No book of this kind can be truly comprehensive, but we believe that we have provided something that may contribute to the other important outcome – an improved quality of life.

# Useful contacts

## General

**Bipolar UK**
Tel.: 020 7931 6480
Website: www.bipolaruk.org.uk

**BootsWebMd**
Website: www.webmd.boots.com
An online service for information about specific drugs and medical conditions.

**British Association for Behavioural and Cognitive Psychotherapies**
Imperial House
Hornby Street
Bury
Lancashire BL9 5BN
Tel.: 0161 705 4304
Website: www.babcp.com

**British Association for Counselling and Psychotherapy**
BACP House
15 St John's Business Park
Lutterworth
Leics LE17 4HB
Tel.: 01455 883300
Website: www.bacp.co.uk

**British Heart Foundation**
Greater London House
180 Hampstead Road
London NW1 7AW
Tel.: 020 7554 0000
For medical information or support: 0300 330 3311
Website: www.bhf.org.uk

**Carers Trust**
32–36 Loman Street
London SE1 0EH
Tel.: 0844 800 4361
Website: www.carers.org

**Carers UK**
20 Great Dover Street
London SE1 4LX
Tel.: 020 7378 4999
Advice line: 0808 808 7777 (free; 10 a.m. to 12 noon, 2 p.m. to 4 p.m.,
Wednesdays and Thursdays)
Website: www.carersuk.org

**Council for Information on Tranquillisers, Antidepressants and
Painkillers (CITAP)** (formerly **CITA**)
Helpline: 0151 932 0102 (10 a.m. to 1 p.m., Monday to Friday, weekends
and bank holidays)
Website: www.citawithdrawal.org.uk

**Crisis**
66 Commercial Street
London E1 6LT
Tel.: 0300 636 1967
Website: www.crisis.org.uk

**Cruse Bereavement Care**
Tel.: 020 8939 9530 (office administration); 0844 477 9400 (daytime
helpline)
Website: www.cruse.org.uk

**Depression Alliance**
20 Great Dover Street
London SE1 4LX
Tel.: 0845 123 23 20
Website: www.depressionalliance.org/

**Depression UK**
c/o Self Help Nottingham
Ormiston House
32–36 Pelham Street
Nottingham NG1 2EG
Website: www.depressionuk.org

**Macmillan Cancer Support**
Tel.: 0808 808 00 00 (support line)
Website: www.macmillan.org.uk

**Making Space**
Lyne House
46 Allen Street
Warrington
Cheshire WA2 7JB
Tel.: 01925 571680
Website: www.makingspace.co.uk
Helps all those with schizophrenia and other forms of mental illness.

**Mind**
15–19 Broadway
London E15 4BQ
Tel.: 020 8519 2122
Info line: 0300 123 3393
Website: www.mind.org.uk
See also **Young Minds**

**NetDoctor** (for online information about drugs and illnesses)
Website: www.netdoctor.co.uk

**NHS Direct**
Tel.: 111 (for health advice and information)
Website: www.nhsdirect.nhs.uk

**Patients Association**
PO Box 935
Harrow
Middlesex HA1 3YJ
Tel.: 020 8423 9111; 0845 608 4455 (helpline)
Website: www.patients-association.com

**Relate**
Tel.: 0300 100 1234
Website: www.relate.org.uk
Assists with relationship matters.

**Rethink Mental Illness**
89 Albert Embankment
London SE1 7TP
Tel.: 0300 5000 927
Website: www.rethink.org
There are also sister charities in Wales (see www.hafal.org) and Northern
Ireland (Mind Wise New Vision; see www.mindwisenv.org).

**Royal College of Psychiatrists**
17 Belgrave Square
London SW1X 8PG
Tel.: 020 7235 2351
Website: www.rcpsych.ac.uk

**Samaritans**
Freepost RSRB-KKYB-CYJK
Chris, PO Box 90 90
Stirling FK8 2SA
National Helpline: 08457 90 90 90 (24 hours a day, 365 days a year; local
rate)
Website: www.samaritans.org.uk
Email: jo@samaritans.org

**SANE**
First Floor, Cityside House
40 Adler Street
London E1 1EE
Tel.: 020 7375 1002
Helpline: 0845 767 8000 (local call rates, 6 p.m. to 11 p.m.)
Website: www.sane.org.uk

**Seasonal Affective Disorder Association**
PO Box 989
Steyning BN44 3HG
Website: www.sada.org.uk

**The Sleep Council**
High Corn Mill
Chapel Hill
Skipton
North Yorkshire BD23 1NL
Tel.: 0845 058 4595 (admin); freephone leaflet line: 0800 018 2923
Website: www.sleepcouncil.org.uk

**Stroke Association**
Tel.: 020 7566 0300 (admin); 0303 3033 100 (helpline)
Website: www.stroke.org.uk

**Survivors' Poetry**
Studio 11, Bickerton House
25–27 Bickerton Road
London N19 5JT
Tel.: 020 7281 4654
Website: www.survivorspoetry.org

**United Kingdom Council for Psychotherapy**
Second Floor, Edward House
2 Wakley Street
London EC1V 7LT
Tel.: 020 7014 9955
Website: www.psychotherapy.org.uk

**Victim Support**
Supportline: 0845 30 30 900
Website: www.victimsupport.org.uk

**Young Minds**
Tel.: 020 7089 5050
Parents' helpline: 0808 802 5544
Website: www.youngminds.org.uk

# Help with debt problems

**Citizens Advice Bureaux (CAB)**
Find your local branch online, or via your local library or GPs' surgery.
National phone service: 08444 111 444 (England); 08444 77 20 20
(Wales).
TextRelay users: 08444 111 445. Note: calls to 08444 numbers cost 5p per
minute from a BT landline and may cost considerably more from mobile
and other phones.
Websites: www.citizensadvice.org.uk *and* www.adviceguide.org.uk

**National Debtline**
Tricorn House
51–53 Hagley Road
Edgbaston
Birmingham B16 8TP
Tel.: 0800 808 4000 (freephone, 9 a.m. to 9 p.m., Monday to Friday; 9.30
a.m. to 1 p.m., Saturday; otherwise leave a message with the 24-hour
voicemail to request an information pack, or send a fax to 0121 410 6230)
Website: www.nationaldebtline.co.uk

**Payplan**
Tel.(from a landline): 0800 280 2816, 8 a.m. to 9 p.m., Monday to Friday;
9 a.m. to 3 p.m. From a mobile it may be cheaper to use 020 7760 8980.
Website: www.payplan.com
For debt help and advice.

**StepChange Debt Charity** (formerly **Consumer Credit Counselling
Service)**
Wade House
Merrion Centre
Leeds LS2 8NG
Tel.: 0800 138 1111 (freephone, including from mobiles); 8 a.m. to 8 p.m.,
Monday to Friday; 9 a.m. to 3 p.m., Saturday).
Website: www.stepchange.org

# Help with alcohol- and drug-related problems, including smoking

Alcoholics Anonymous
Registered Office
PO Box 1
10 Toft Green
York YO1 7NJ
National helpline: 0845 769 7555 (24-hour; confidential)
Website: www.alcoholics-anonymous.org.uk

**Al-Anon**
Tel.: 020 7403 0888 (confidential helpline, 10 a.m. to 10 p.m., 365 days a year)
Website: www.al-anonuk.org.uk
Offers understanding and support for families and friends of problem drinkers.

**Cocaine Anonymous UK**
CAUK Talbot House
204–226 Imperial Way
Rayners Lane
Harrow
Middlesex HA2 7HH
Tel.: 0800 612 0225 (10 a.m. to 10 p.m., daily; free from landlines)
Website: www.cauk.org.uk

**Drinkline**
Tel.: 0800 917 8282 (Freephone; 9 a.m. to 8 p.m., Monday to Friday; weekends 11 a.m. to 4 p.m.)
This national alcohol helpline provides a confidential service offering information and support to callers, and to their relatives and friends.

**QUIT**
Quitline: 0800 00 22 00 (free)
Website: www.quit.org.uk
Email: stopsmoking@quit.org.uk (counselling)

# References

American Psychiatric Association (2013). *Diagnostic and Statistical Manual of Mental Disorders*, 5th ed. (DSM-5). Arlington, VA.

Andrew, A., Knapp, M., McCrone, P., Parsonage, M. and Trachtenberg, M. (2012). *Effective Interventions in Schizophrenia: The Economic Case. A report prepared for the Schizophrenia Commission*. London School of Economics Personal Social Services Research Unit. <http://www.lse.ac.uk/LSEHealthAndSocialCare/pdf/LSE-economic-report-FINAL-12-Nov.pdf>.

Branch, R. and Willson, R. (2010). *Cognitive Behaviour Therapy for Dummies*, 2nd ed. Chichester, UK: John Wiley & Sons.

Kapur, S. (2003). 'Psychosis as a state of aberrant salience: A framework linking biology, phenomenology and pharmacology in schizophrenia'. *American Journal of Psychiatry* 160(1): 13–23.

Kuipers, E., Leff, J. and Lam, D. (2002). *Family Work for Schizophrenia: A Practical Guide*. London: Gaskell Press.

Leucht, S., Corves, C., Arbter, D., Engel, R. R., Li, C. and Davis, J. M. (2009). 'Second-generation versus first-generation antipsychotic drugs for schizophrenia: A meta-analysis'. *Lancet* 373(9657): 31–41.

McManus, S., Meltzer, H. and Campion, J. (2010). *Cigarette Smoking and Mental Health in England: Data from the Adult Psychiatric Morbidity Survey 2007*. London: National Centre for Social Research.

Royal College of Psychiatrists (2012). *Report of the National Audit of Schizophrenia (NAS) 2012*. London: Healthcare Quality Improvement Partnership. <www.rcpsych.ac.uk/workinpsychiatry/qualityimprovement/nationalclinicalaudits/schizophrenia/nationalschizophreniaaudit.aspx>.

Taylor, D., Paton, C. and Kapur, S. (Eds) (2012). *The Maudsley Prescribing Guidelines in Psychiatry*, 11th ed. Chichester, UK: Wiley-Blackwell.

The Schizophrenia Commission (2012). *The Abandoned Illness: A Report from the Schizophrenia Commission*. London: Rethink Mental Illness. <www.schizophreniacommission.org.uk>.

Thornicroft, G., Szmukler, G., Mueser, K. T. and Drake, R. E. (Eds) (2011). *Oxford Textbook of Community Mental Health*. Oxford: Oxford University Press.

Ussher, M., Stanbury, L., Cheeseman, V. and Faulkner, G. (2007). 'Physical activity preferences and perceived barriers to activity among persons with severe mental illness in the United Kingdom'. *Psychiatric Services* 58(3):405–8.

van der Gaag, M., Stant, A., Wolters, K., Buskens, E. and Wiersma, D. (2011). 'Cognitive-behavioural therapy for persistent and recurrent psychosis in people with schizophrenia-spectrum disorder: Cost-effectiveness analysis'. *British Journal of Psychiatry* 198(1): 59–65.

Varase, F., Smeets, F., Drukker, M. *et al.* (2012). 'Childhood adversities increase the risk of psychosis: A meta-analysis of patient-control, prospective- and cross-sectional cohort studies'. *Schizophrenia Bulletin* 38(4):661–71.

Veale, D. and Willson, R. (2007). *Manage Your Mood: How to Use Behavioural Activation Techniques to Overcome Depression*. London: Constable & Robinson.

Whitfield, G. and Davidson, A. (2007). *Cognitive Behavioural Therapy Explained*. Milton Keynes, UK: Radcliffe Publishing.

World Health Organization (2010). *The International Statistical Classification of Diseases and Health Related Problems*, revision 10 (ICD-10). Geneva: World Health Organization.

Yusuf, S., Hawken, S., Ounpuu, S. *et al.* (2004). 'Effect of potentially modifiable risk factors associated with myocardial infarction in 52 countries (the INTERHEART study): Case-control study'. *Lancet* 364(9438): 937–52.

# Index